Sepsis

New Strategies for Management

T0238575

Jordi Rello • Marcos I. Restrepo

Editors

Sepsis

New Strategies for Management

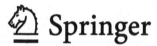
Springer

Jordi Rello, MD, PhD
Critical Care Department – Joan XXIII
University Hospital
Universidad Rovira & Virgili
and Institut Pere Virgili
CIBER Enfermedades Respiratorias
Doctor Mallafre Guasch, 4, 43007
Tarragona, Spain
jrello.hj23.ics@gencat.net

Marcos I. Restrepo, MD, MSc
Division Pulmonary and Critical Care
Medicine
San Antonio, TX 78229-4404, USA

Department of Medicine
University of Texas Health Science
Center at San Antonio
San Antonio, TX, USA

Veterans Evidence-Based Research
Dissemination Implementation Center
(VERDICT)
South Texas Veterans Health Care System
Audie L. Murphy Division
7400 Merton Minter Blvd (11C6)
San Antonio, TX 78229-4404, USA
restrepom@uthscsa.edu

ISBN   978-3-642-09782-9   e-ISBN   978-3-540-79001-3

DOI:10.1007/978-3-540-79001-3

Cover design: eStudio Calamar Steinen, Barcelona

Printed on acid-free paper

9 8 7 6 5 4 3 2 1

springer.com

Preface

Infectious-related mortality has remained an important problem around the world, and the majority of these deaths are related to pneumonia and sepsis. Although new interventions have emerged over the last decade, the mortality rates for these illnesses have remained significantly high and represent an important health care problem. This book is intended to address new concepts in medical care for a wide variety of clinicians who are involved in the care of patients with pneumonia and sepsis. This material is a compendium that goes from basic science research regarding genetics in sepsis and the impact of inflammation and aging in pneumococcal disease to new and future interventions translating basic information into clinical practice. Other topics covered in this book include issues regarding antibiotic therapy, such as other roles for macrolides, and appropriate dose adjustment and pharmacodynamic considerations. Finally, a wide variety of novel and innovative therapies are reviewed, including corticosteroids, statins, and nonspecific removal of sepsis mediators that are being used in patients with pneumonia and sepsis.

An outstanding panel of international experts has focused on recent developments. It has been an honor working with them, and thanks to their efforts the bulk of the references are less than five years old. Ms. Rosi Luque, with the sponsorship of the CIBERes, helped us in the coordination of the editorial work, and we are indebted to her for this. The authors hope that their experiences as summarized in these pages are of value to the reader and, ultimately, improve the care of patients with pneumonia and sepsis.

Jordi Rello   Tarragona, Spain
Marcos I. Restrepo   San Antonio, TX

Contents

Contributors

Carlos Agustí
Pneumology Service, Hospital Clínic de Barcelona, C/Villarroel, 170,
08036 Barcelona, Spain
cagusti@clinic.ub.es

Antonio Anzueto
Department of Medicine, University of Texas Health Science Center,
7400 Merton Minter Blvd (111 East), San Antonio, TX 78229-4404, USA
Anzueto@Uthscsa.Edu

Robert Boots
Department of Intensive Care Medicine, Royal Brisbane and Women's Hospitals,
Herston, QLD 4029, Australia
r.boots@mailbox.uq.edu.au

Xosé Luis Pérez-Fernandez
Critical Care Department – Hospital Universitari de Bellvitge
Feixa Llarga, s/n 08907 – Hospitalet de Llobregat (Barcelona), Spain
josep@csub.scs.es

Jeffrey Lipman
Anaesthesiology and Critical Care, University of Queensland, Brisbane, Australia
Department of Intensive Care Medicine, Royal Brisbane and Women's Hospitals,
Herston, QLD 4029, Australia
j.lipman@uq.edu.au

Mónica Magret
Critical Care Department – Joan XXIII University Hospital, Doctor Mallafre
Guasch, 4, 43007 Tarragona, Spain
mnicamgrt@yahoo.es

Rafael Mañez
Critical Care Department, Bellvitge University Hospital, Feixa Llarga, s/n 08907
Hospitalet de Llobregat (Barcelona), Spain
rmanez@csub.scs.es

Eric M. Mortensen
Department of Medicine, University of Texas Health Science Center
at San Antonio, San Antonio, TX, USA
VERDICT/South Texas Veterans Health Care System, Audie L. Murphy
Division, Ambulatory Care (11C6), 7400 Merton Minter Boulevard, San Antonio,
TX 78284, USA
mortensene@uthscsa.edu

Carlos J. Orihuela
Department of Microbiology and Immunology, The University of Texas Health
Science Center at San Antonio, Mail Code 7758, 7703 Floyd Curl Drive,
San Antonio, TX 78229-3900, USA
orihuela@uthscsa.edu

Jordi Rello
Critical Care Department – Joan XXIII University Hospital, Universidad Rovira
& Virgili and Institut Pere Virgili, CIBER Enfermedades Respiratorias, Doctor
Mallafre Guasch, 4, 43007 Tarragona, Spain
jrello.hj23.ics@gencat.net

Marcos I. Restrepo
Division Pulmonary and Critical Care Medicine, San Antonio, TX 78229-4404,
USA
Department of Medicine, University of Texas Health Science Center
at San Antonio, San Antonio, TX, USA
Veterans Evidence-Based Research Dissemination Implementation Center
(VERDICT), South Texas Veterans Health Care System, Audie L. Murphy
Division, 7400 Merton Minter Blvd (11C6), San Antonio, TX 78229-4404, USA
restrepom@uthscsa.edu

Jason Roberts
Burns Trauma and Critical Care Research Centre, Level 3 Ned Hanlon
Building, Royal Brisbane and Women's Hospital, Herston, QLD 4029, Australia
j.roberts2@uq.edu.au

Alejandro Rodríguez
Critical Care Department – Joan XXIII University Hospital, CIBER Enfermedades
Respiratorias, Doctor Mallafre Guasch, 4, 43007 Tarragona, Spain
ahr1161@yahoo.es, Arodri.hj23.ics@gencat.net

Angela J. Rodriguez
Department of Medicine, The University of Texas Health Science Center at San
Antonio, Mail Code 7758, 7703 Floyd Curl Drive, San Antonio, TX 77229-3900,
USA
rodrigueza12@uthscsa.edu

Joan Sabater Riera
Critical Care Department – Hospital Universitari de Bellvitge
Feixa Llarga, s/n 08907 – Hospitalet de Llobregat (Barcelona), Spain
jsabater@csub.scs.es

Oriol Sibila
Pneumology Service, Hospital Universitari Son Dureta, Fundació Caubet-Cimera,
Andrea Dòria 55, 07014 Palma de Mallorca, Illes Balears, Spain
osibila@hsd.es

Antoni Torres
Cap de Servei de Pneumologia i Alzlèrgia Respiratòria, Hospital Clínic de
Barcelona, C/Villarroel, 170, 08036 Barcelona, Spain
atorres@ub.edu

Andrew Udy
Department of Intensive Care Medicine, Royal Brisbane and Women's Hospitals,
Herston, QLD 4029, Australia
andrew_udy@health.qld.gov.au

Grant W. Waterer
School of Medicine and Pharmacology, University of Western Australia, Australia
Department of Respiratory Medicine, Royal Perth Hospital, Australia
waterer@cyllene.uwa.edu.au

Richard G. Wunderink
Pulmonary and Critical Care Division
Northwestern University Feinberg
School of Medicine, Chicago, Illinois, 60611, USA
r-wunderink@northwestern.edu

Chapter 1
Macrolides in Severe Community-Acquired Pneumonia and Sepsis

Marcos I. Restrepo, Eric M. Mortensen, Grant W. Waterer,
Richard G. Wunderink, and Antonio Anzueto

1.1 Introduction

More than 750,000 cases of severe sepsis occur annually (Angus et al. 2001), making the incidence of severe sepsis higher than that of breast cancer, AIDS, or first myocardial infarction. The incidence of sepsis is increasing because of the aging population, the growing number of immunocompromised patients, and the increasing use of invasive procedures, and to a lesser extent, because of antibiotic resistance among pathogens. In the United States alone, almost $17 billion is spent each year treating patients with sepsis (Angus et al. 2001).

Despite advances in care, more than 210,000 patients with severe sepsis die annually (Angus et al. 2001). The mortality rate associated with severe sepsis remains between 20% and 80% (Zeni et al. 1997). Even dysfunction of a single organ places patients at a significant risk for dying (about 20%), with mortality rates increasing approximately 15–20% for each additional dysfunctional organ (Vincent et al. 1998). Mortality rates are highest (ranging from 50 to 80%) for patients with cardiovascular compromise (septic shock) (Rangel-Frausto et al. 1995). Respiratory infections, whether community- or hospital-acquired account for the most sepsis cases (Angus et al. 2001; Bernard et al. 2001; Martin et al. 2003). Community-acquired pneumonia (CAP) is one the most common reasons for sepsis and is itself, independent of sepsis, the seventh leading cause of death and the leading cause of infectious death in the United States (Hoyert et al. 2005).

The pathogenesis of sepsis is complex and, despite significant advances, still not well understood (Annane et al. 2005). Essentially, sepsis is the result of the interaction between microorganisms and/or their products and the host factors released in response (cytokines and other mediators). An important component of the host response is the initial innate mechanisms developed to protect the organism from harm. However, in sepsis, the immune response itself initiates a cascade of secondary responses that may lead to organ dysfunction and even death, despite eradication of the invading microorganism. Initial concepts of sepsis as an uncontrolled proinflammatory response have been replaced by more complex models, which also incorporate dysregulation of anti-inflammatory, coagulation, and tissue healing/repair pathways (Annane et al. 2005). However, the proinflammatory response,

J. Rello, M.I. Restrepo (eds.) *Sepsis: New Strategies for Management.*
doi:10.1007/978-3-540-79001-3 © Springer-Verlag 2008

particularly release of tumor necrosis factor (TNFα), is clearly critical in the early phase of sepsis (Van Amersfoort et al. 2003; Annane et al. 2005; Carlson et al. 2005; van Leeuwen et al. 2005).

Normally, a potent complex immunologic cascade ensures a prompt protective response to microbial invasion in humans. A deficient immunologic defense may allow infection to become established; however, an excessive or poorly regulated response may harm the host through a maladaptive release of endogenously generated inflammatory compounds. The complexity of immunologic defenses makes the development of pharmacologic interventions difficult (Parrillo et al. 1990). A key element associated with early biochemical events in sepsis is cytokines, which are host-produced, pleomorphic immunoregulatory peptides. The most widely investigated cytokines are tumor necrosis factor (TNFα), interleukin-1 (IL-1), IL-6, IL-8, which are generally proinflammatory, and IL-1Ra and IL-10, which tend to be antiinflammatory. A trigger, such as microbial toxin, stimulates the production of TNFα and IL-1, which in turn promote endothelial cell-leukocyte adhesion, release of proteases and arachidonate metabolites, and activation of clotting. IL-1 and TNFα are synergistic and share some biologic effects, and their inhibition improves organ function and survival in animal models of sepsis. IL-8, a neutrophil chemotaxin, may have an especially important role in perpetuating tissue inflammation. IL-1Ra and IL-10, which are perhaps counterregulatory, inhibit the generation of TNFα, augment the action of acute-phase reactants and immunoglobulins, and inhibit T-lymphocyte and macrophage production. TNFα is a cytokine that, for a number of reasons, is thought to play a central role in the pathogenesis of sepsis and septic shock: (1) TNFα concentrations are increased during clinical and experimental sepsis (Debets et al. 1989; Dofferhoff et al. 1992; Casey et al. 1993); (2) increasing concentrations and especially persistence of high concentrations of TNFα during sepsis are associated with decreased survival (Dofferhoff et al. 1992); (3) endotoxin and bacterial challenge in animals and low-grade endotoxinchallenge in humans lead to TNFα release (Michie et al. 1988); (4) TNFα challenge in animals (Eichenholz et al. 1992) and humans (Creaven et al. 1989; Lenk et al. 1989) leads to or simulates sepsis and organ failure; and (5) TNFα neutralization in experimental sepsis frequently leads to amelioration of sepsis symptoms and increases survival (Beutler et al. 1985; Tracey et al. 1987; Beutler 1993). These studies clearly underline the pivotal role that TNFα plays in the pathogenesis of sepsis.

Based on the findings of the studies outlined above, drugs against TNFα were produced and clinical trials were conducted to test whether inhibiting TNFα also improves survival in human sepsis. Early studies of anti-TNFα antibodies and TNFα-receptor fusion proteins did not lead to the results hoped for in phase III trials (Abraham et al. 1995, 1997, 1998; Cohen and Carlet 1996; Fisher et al. 1996; Reinhart et al. 1996). However, a meta-analysis of all randomized controlled clinical studies shows that anti-TNFα strategies with monoclonal antibodies are effective in increasing survival, with a mean improvement in survival of ~3% (Reinhart and Karzai 2001). It is striking that most trials showed a small, albeit nonsignificant, increase in survival in patients treated with anti-TNFα drugs, suggesting that TNFα inhibition has led to beneficial effects in subgroups of patients. The recent positive results with afelimomab targeting patients with sepsis and elevated serum inter-leukin-6 levels (Panacek et al. 2004) further reinforces the fact that effective reduc-tion in TNFα production or effect has therapeutic potential.

A variety of reasons have been suggested for why the effects of these anti-TNFα strategies have not produced the dramatic clinical benefit expected from the animal studies (Reinhart and Karzai 2001; Eichacker et al. 2002; Deans et al. 2005). In addition to other reasons, each of these strategies attempted to neutralize already-produced TNFα. A more effective strategy may be to suppress or modulate the ongoing production of TNFα and the other cytokines. In addition, each of these strategies affects the intravascular space predominantly, if not exclusively. Much of the organ dysfunction caused by sepsis may be occurring in spaces without direct intravascular involvement, such as the respiratory epithelium. In addition, the effect of anti-TNFα antibodies is only on extracellular or membrane-associated TNFα and not at intracellular levels (Fumeaux et al. 2004).

Early in the antibiotic era, the inability of appropriate antibiotic therapy to sal-vage all patients with severe infections was recognized. The classic example was and remains penicillin treatment of bacteremic pneumococcal pneumonia. However, Mortensen and colleagues showed that early appropriate guideline concordant therapy may improve survival in hospitalized patients with community-acquired pneumonia even in the first 48 h of admission (Mortensen et al. 2006b). More modern critical care has focused on organ support, such as early aggressive fluid resuscita-tion, lung-protective ventilatory strategies, and renal replacement therapy. Once again, while beneficial, a significant percent (20–30%) of severe sepsis patients die despite this state-of-the-art care.

1.2 Immunomodulation in Sepsis

Immunomodulation was thought to be an important mechanism to improve outcome of sepsis. While still logical and strongly supported by animal models, the results of these interventions have been disappointing. The early focus was on anti-TNFα strategies because of pivotal role in animal models of sepsis (Beutler et al. 1985; Tracey et al. 1987). However, these studies, despite encouraging preliminary studies or subgroup results, did not demonstrate an overall improvement in 28-day mortality (Abraham et al. 1995, 2001). Subsequent ones focusing on other mediators, such as IL-1 receptor antagonist, had similar results (Eichacker et al. 2002; Panacek et al. 2004). Whether low dose steroids have a benefit via replacement of relative adrenal insufficiency (Annane et al. 2002) or its immunomodulatory benefit is unclear.

The first immunomodulatory agent specifically approved by the Food and Drug Administration (FDA) for use in severe sepsis was drotrecogin-alfa activated, based on its overall 6.1% absolute risk reduction in a large Phase III trial (Bernard et al. 2001). Subsequent questions have arisen regarding the efficacy of drotrecogin-alfa activated for patients at low risk of dying (Abraham et al. 2005), with infections other than pneumonia (Abraham et al. 2005; Laterre et al. 2005), and its overall risk/benefit (Eichacker et al. 2005). The cost (exceeded $7,000), the adverse effects (bleeding), and the limited efficacy to those severely ill with an acute physiologic and chronic health assessment (APACHE)-II score of ≥25 and several organ failures have limited the use in clinical practice.

The conclusion is that new immunomodulatory agents with either greater efficacy or lower toxicity are clearly needed. A variety of agents are presently in clinical trials. However, most are new molecular compounds which are likely to be similarly expensive to drotrecogin-alfa activated and may have significant or unknown side effects or toxicity. The potential to use a macrolide antibiotic, with its known side-effect profile and low cost, is particularly attractive.

1.3   Macrolides as Immunomodulators

The macrolides are a class of antibiotics that are characterized by a many-membered macrocyclic lactone ring. The original antibiotic was erythromycin, which was found to be a metabolic product of *Streptomyces erythreus*. Other common members of the class include roxithromycin, clarithromycin, and azithromycin. Azithromycin is derived from erythromycin by having a methyl-substituted nitrogen in its 15-member lactone ring. Macrolides with 15-member and 14-member lactone rings (roxithromycin, clarithromycin, and erythromycin) appear to have immunomodulatory properties that the larger macrolides do not have (Yamanaka et al. 2001). The macrolide antibiotics are structurally similar to the macrolide immunosuppressant agents' tacrolimus and rapamycin.

The antimicrobial mechanism of action of macrolide antibiotics is to inhibit bacterial protein synthesis by reversibly binding to the 50S ribosomal subunit, blocking transpeptidation and/or translocation in susceptible organisms. It is suggested that macrolides have immunomodulatory benefits that are independent of their bactericidal/bacteriostatic properties. The following data supporting these effects of macrolides derive from laboratory, animal, and clinical studies.

1.4   Laboratory Evidence

A considerable number of in vitro and in vivo studies have documented immunomodulatory properties of macrolides. The effect of macrolides on inflammatory molecules is confusing and somewhat variable. Macrolide antibiotics fairly consistently reduce production of inflammatory cytokines, including TNFα, IL-1β, IL-6, IL-8, and gamma interferon (IFN-γ) (Vazifeh et al. 2000) (summarized in Table 1.1).

The effect of macrolides may be somewhat dose dependent. Macrolides also appear to decrease intercellular adhesion molecule (ICAM)-1 (Khair et al. 1995; Kawasaki et al. 1998), although the effect of this on polymorphonuclear (PMNs) leukocytes recruitment into the lung is inconclusive. Macrolides are consistently

Table 1.1 Macrolide effect on cell lines

Cell line	Effect
Neutrophils	• Increase apoptosis
	• Decrease oxidants
Respiratory epithelial cells	• Increase IL-6 and IL-8 levels
T lymphocytes	• Decrease IL-1 and TNF levels
	• Increase IL-2, IL-4, and IFN-gamma
Monocytes	• Decrease IL-1, TNF, and GM-CSF
	• Increase IL-8 and IL-10 levels

GM-CSF granulocyte-macrophage colony-stimulating factor; *IFN* interferon; *IL* interleukin; *TNF* tumor necrosis factor

shown to suppress nitric oxide release, probably via inhibition of inducible nitric oxide synthetase (iNOS) gene expression (Tamaoki 2004). However, macrolides appear to increase neutrophil degranulation as measured by ex vivo release of bactericidal/permeability increasing protein (BPI), neutrophil elastase, and lactoferrin (Schultz et al. 2000). At the same time, they reduce IL-8 levels and other chemokines levels. In both human respiratory epithelial cells (Desaki et al. 2000) and monocytes (Kikuchi et al. 2002), macrolides appear to suppress nuclear factor kappa beta activation. A suggestion that the anti-inflammatory action of macrolides may be upstream of cytokine action (Vazifeh et al. 2000) remains highly speculative. The effect of macrolides may vary and could be cell-type specific. Immunomodulatory effects have been studied in neutrophils (Vazifeh et al. 2000), monocytes/macrophages (Khan et al. 1999; Kohri et al. 2000; Kikuchi et al. 2002), keratinocytes (Kobayashi et al. 2004), and respiratory epithelial cells (Desaki et al. 2000). Erythromycin inhibited IL-8 production in response to *Pseudomonas* stimulation in neutrophils but not alveolar macrophages (Oishi et al. 1994). Given the multitude of effects, macrolides likely act at multiple sites within the inflammatory cascade (Tamaoki 2004). Macrolides readily diffuse into intracellular sites and accumulate in cells at up to 50 times the serum concentration (Ishiguro et al. 1989; Rodvold 1999; Beringer et al. 2005), and interference with multiple target sites is quite feasible.

Macrolides have other important non-antibiotic properties relevant to sepsis. Firstly, macrolides inhibit neutrophil oxidative function, possibly by interference with the phospholipase D-phosphatidate phosphohydrolase transduction pathway (Abdelghaffar et al. 1997), or via protein kinase A inhibition (Mitsuyama et al. 1995). In addition, macrolides reduce respiratory secretions (Tamaoki 2004) by an undetermined mechanism. While potentially important, these effects do not explain macrolide inhibition of cytokine production and need further evaluation.

1.5 Experimental Evidence

Two recent publications have demonstrated a clear survival advantage of clarithromycin in a rabbit-pyelonephritis model of sepsis (Giamarellos-Bourboulis et al. 2005a,b). Although clarithromycin had no antimicrobial activity against the *Escherichia coli* causing the sepsis, its addition to therapy resulted in a marked increase in survival. The survival benefit was almost equivalent to that of an active gram-negative bactericidal agent (amikacin). Furthermore, the increase in survival with administration of clarithromycin was accompanied by a marked decrease in monocyte activation and TNFα production compared to control (Giamarellos-Bourboulis et al. 2005a,b). Earlier work by the same group showed a similar benefit in a rabbit *Pseudomonas*-peritonitis sepsis model (Giamarellos-Bourboulis et al. 2004), demonstrating that the effect was dependent on neither site nor microorganism.

The strong association between TNFα and severe sepsis led to Phase II and III trials of anti-TNFα agents with different blocking strategies. One possible explanation for the lack of a beneficial effect of these agents was that a balance of positive and negative effects of blocking the TNFα response, rather than lack of efficacy alone, was responsible (Bone 1996; Reinhart and Karzai 2001). Macrolides have a significant anti-inflammatory action, reducing TNFα by up to fourfold but not completely ablating TNFα response (Khan et al. 1999; Kohri et al. 2000; Vazifeh et al. 2000; Kikuchi et al. 2002; Kobayashi et al. 2004). Modulation rather than complete ablation of TNFα may avoid many of the deleterious effects of anti-TNFα antibodies including increased risk of nosocomial infections. Furthermore, as TNFα response also involves autocrine signaling in some cell types (Kuno et al. 2005; Vila-del Sol and Fresno 2005), there are potential advantages of macrolides over anti-TNFα antibodies as the former have an intracellular (presecretory) mechanism of action. In addition, not all cytokines are affected equally by macrolides. Fluoroquinolones also have immunomodulatory effects (Dalhoff and Shalit 2003; Hall et al. 2004; Williams et al. 2005). When PMNs leukocytes from healthy volunteers were stimulated with phorbol myristate acetate, clarithromycin decreased IL-4 expression but did not affect the Th1 cytokine IFN-γ, whereas fluoroquinolones suppressed both IL-4 and IFN-γ (Williams et al. 2005). The net result was that the Th1/Th2 ratio increased with clarithromycin, potentially maintaining protection from a bacterial challenge (Ferguson et al. 1999).

Finally, it is clear that macrolides alter the production of a much wider range of inflammatory proteins than just TNFα, providing additional potential beneficial responses in patients with severe sepsis.

1.6 Clinical Evidence

Macrolide antibiotics have been used as antimicrobial agents for more than 50 years. More recently, clinicians have begun to use these agents not for their antimicrobial action but for their effect on immune function. The most dramatic example of the efficacy of macrolides as immune modulators is in diffuse panbronchiolitis. This noninfectious, autoimmune lung condition had a 70% 5-year mortality rate until long-term low-dose erythromycin was found to reduce the 5-year mortality rate to <20% (Yamamoto et al. 1990; Kudoh et al. 1998; Kadota et al. 2003).

Table 1.2 Macrolide effects on different respiratory conditions in human subjects

Conditions	Effects
Asthma	Increase FEV_1, change on the provocative dose of methacoline
Bronchiolitis obliterans	Increase FEV_1, decrease neutrophil and IL-8 levels
Cryptogenic pneumonia	Symptomatic improvement and radiographic resolution
Cystic fibrosis	Increase FEV_1, reduced risk of bacterial exacerbation and reduced need for antimicrobial therapy
Diffuse panbronchiolitis	Improve survival, decrease sputum production, increase FEV_1 and vital capacity
COPD	Decrease IL-8, TNFα, lactoferrin, and 2-microglobulin of neutrophils

COPD chronic obstructive pulmonary disease; *FEV_1* forced expiratory volume in the first second; *IL*, interleukin; *TNF* tumor necrosis factor

The exact mechanism is unknown but is clearly not solely antimicrobial (Amsden 2005). Macrolide antibiotics are now being used in a variety of predominantly respiratory diseases as immunomodulatory agents. Some are clearly infectious, such as cystic fibrosis (Equi et al. 2002; Hoiby 2002; Wolter et al. 2002a,b; Saiman et al. 2003; Schultz 2004; Southern and Barker 2004; Amsden 2005; Clement et al. 2006) and bronchiectasis (Koh et al. 1997; Yalcin et al. 2006) (Table 1.2). In these cases, other effects, such as inhibition of bacterial toxic or biofilm production, quorum sensing, and even intracellular killing despite resistance of the bacteria by usual sensitivity testing, may explain the beneficial effect. However, an immunomodulatory role has been suggested by an analysis of cytokine levels and a differential response with other antibiotics.

Other disorders where macrolides have been suggested to be of benefit are clearly not infectious (Table 1.2). In obliterative bronchiolitis post transplant (Gerhardt et al. 2003; Schultz 2004; Tamaoki et al. 2004; Stover and Mangino 2005; Verleden et al. 2006), they appear to have significant efficacy. Other disorders in which macrolides have been suggested to be effective include asthma (Miyatake et al. 1991a,b; Hendeles 1992; Amayasu et al. 2000; Kraft et al. 2002; Gotfried 2004; Hatipoglu and Rubinstein 2004; Kostadima et al. 2004; Amsden 2005; Johnston et al. 2006; Piacentini et al. 2007), chronic obstructive pulmonary disease (Culic et al. 2002; Basyigit et al. 2004; Parnham et al. 2005), pyometra (Mikamo et al. 1998), and even as a post operative anti-inflammatory analgesic (Chow et al. 2000).

However, the strongest data available is derived from clinical studies in patients with pneumococcal and community-acquired pneumonia (CAP). Interest in the role of macrolides as immunomodulatory agents for sepsis was first stimulated by the retrospective review of mortality in bacteremic pneumococcal community-acquired pneumonia done by Waterer and collaborators (Waterer et al. 2001). The use of a single effective antibiotic was associated with an increased mortality compared to the use of two effective agents. The two populations were well matched for severity, as suggested by APACHE II scores and pneumonia severity index score. Macrolide-containing combinations were the most common type of combination therapy and had lower mortality than predicted by the APACHE II prediction model. The statistically significant mortality difference persisted in multivariate analysis. When only patients with PSI scores >90 (potential ICU patients (Mandell et al. 2003)) were analyzed, the predicted mortality-adjusted odds ratio for death with monotherapy was 5.5 (95% confidence interval (CI) 1.7–17.5). Mufson and Stanek (1999) had also documented a significant mortality benefit of adding specifically a macrolide to β-lactam therapy in a large prospective observational trial of bacteremic pneumococcal CAP. Stimulated by these results, two large prospective observational trials (Martinez et al. 2003; Baddour et al. 2004) and a retrospective single site study (Weiss et al. 2004) have all documented a survival advantage to adding a macrolide to a β-lactam for bacteremic pneumococcal infections (Table 1.3).

Table 1.3 Studies of macrolide therapy in patients with serious infections

Reference	Year	Design	Subjects	Infectious disease	Main results
Mufson	1999	Population-based, retrospective cohort	600	Bacteremic pneumococcal pneumonia	Mortality difference among macrolide combination therapy vs. nonmacrolide monotherapy (7.3% vs. 24.2%)
					Absolute risk reduction of 16.9
Waterer	2001	Multicenter, retrospective cohort	225	Bacteremic pneumococcal pneumonia	Mortality difference among macrolide combination therapy vs. nonmacrolide monotherapy (4.4% vs. 19.4%)
					Absolute risk reduction of 15.0
Martinez	2003	Multicenter, prospective cohort	409	Bacteremic pneumococcal pneumonia	In-hospital mortality was lower with macrolide therapy (OR 0.40; 95% CI 0.17–0.92; $p = 0.03$)
Baddour	2004	Multicenter, prospective cohort	844	Bacteremic pneumococcal pneumonia	14-day mortality was lower with combination therapy vs. monotherapy in critically ill patients (23.4% vs. 55.3%; $p = 0.0015$) and ICU-admitted patients (8.2% vs. 23.1%; $p = 0.03$)
					14-day mortality was lower with macrolide therapy (14.6%; $p = 0.007$)

(continued)

Table 1.3 (continued)

Reference	Year	Design	Subjects	Infectious disease	Main results
Weiss	2004	Population based, retrospective cohort	95	Bacteremic pneumococcal infection	Mortality was lower with combination therapy vs. mono-therapy (7.5% vs. 25.6%; $p = 0.002$) with an absolute risk reduction of 18.1
Garcia Vasquez	2005	Multicenter, prospective cohort	1,391	CAP	Mortality was lower with combination therapy vs. mono-therapy in all CAP patients (6.9% vs. 13.3%; $p = 0.001$) and in PSI V patients (25.7% vs. 32.6%; $p = 0.02$)
					Mortality was higher if macrolide therapy was not used (OR 2.95; 95% CI 1.24–3.23)
Rodriguez	2007	Multicenter, prospective cohort	270	ICU CAP with septic shock	28-day ICU survival was higher with combination therapy in CAP patients with shock (HR 1.69; 95% CI 1.09–2.60, $p = 0.01$) and in patients that received macrolide therapy (HR 1.73; 95% CI 1.08–2.76, $p = 0.02$)
Metersky	2007	Population based, retrospective cohort	2,209	Bacteremic pneumonia	Macrolide therapy was associated with lower in-hospital mortality (OR 0.59; 95% CI 0.40–0.88, $p = 0.01$), 30-day mortality (OR 0.61; 95% CI 0.43–0.87, $p = 0.007$) and hospital re-admission within 30 days post discharge (OR 0.59; 95% CI 0.42–0.85, $p = 0.004$)

CAP community-acquired pneumonia; *CI* confidence interval; *HR* hazard ratio; *OR* odds ratio; *PSI* pneumonia severity index

Further support for the addition of macrolides has come from observational studies in more general CAP cohorts which have also documented outcome benefits of combination therapy over monotherapy, especially with β-lactam monotherapy (Dudas et al. 2000; Houck et al. 2001; Brown et al. 2003; Garcia Vazquez et al. 2005). The majority of combination therapy in these studies included a macrolide. These results suggest that the benefit of macrolides may not be limited to bacteremic pneumococcal disease or even to only pneumococcal CAP.

The mortality benefit from the addition of a macrolide appears to be quite striking, with odds ratios for death ranging from 0.22 to 0.45. The greatest difference appears to be in the critically ill with the highest adjusted odds ratios of death without macrolide therapy in the most critically ill as defined by Pittsburgh Bacteremia score (Baddour et al. 2004), PSI score (Waterer et al. 2001), or simply need for ICU care. The survival advantage of macrolides was only apparent when adjusted for severity of illness but was independent of septic shock (Martinez et al. 2003).

The survival curves in all the studies indicate that the mortality reduction consistently begins 48–72 h after the commencement of therapy, with most benefit being seen in the first 7–10 days. These survival curves are representative of all the other studies as well. The timing of the mortality benefit is important, as macrolides appear to be affecting outcome in the initial 2–7-day period when proinflammatory-driven secondary organ failure (such as acute respiratory distress syndrome, renal, and hepatic failure) is the predominant cause of death. The absence of a clearly discernable survival benefit in the first 24–48 h is not unexpected, given the historical data demonstrating that antibiotics have no impact on mortality compared to placebo (or even immune serum) during that period (Austrian and Gold 1964). Patients who die during the first 48 h typically present in refractory septic shock with multiorgan failure already present, markedly limiting the potential for any intervention to affect outcome. However, recent data suggested that empiric guideline concordant antibiotic therapy was associated with lower mortality even during the first 48 h of admission to the hospital in patients with CAP (Mortensen et al. 2006b).

Two principal explanations have been put forward for the observed beneficial effect of macrolides. The first is the already-discussed immunomodulatory properties of macrolides. The second possibility is unrecognized coinfection (in the case of pneumococcal pneumonia) with a second "atypical" pathogen such as *Mycoplasma, Legionella*, or *Chlamydia* (Waterer 2003). However, fluoroquinolones should have been equivalent to, if not better than, macrolides and yet in our study fluoroquinolone monotherapy had worse outcome compared to macrolide combination therapy (Waterer et al. 2001). Several studies only analyzed macrolides provided in the first 48 h (Waterer et al. 2001) and a short course is less likely to result in a mortality difference even if copathogens were present. In addition, the incidence of atypical copathogens is significantly less common in patients with severe CAP requiring ICU admission than in patients hospitalized on a general floor or treated as outpatients (Ruiz et al. 1999).

However, the most convincing data that coverage of atypical pathogens is not the explanation for the survival benefit of macrolides is recent data from Mortensen and colleagues. We have shown that the combination of a β-lactam and a fluoroquinolone is substantially inferior to that of a β-lactam and a macrolide in patients with severe CAP (Mortensen et al. 2006a). The actual mortality in patients receiving macrolide combination therapy was 17.2%, an absolute risk reduction of 13.8% for the general population. Once again, the benefit of a nonquinolone (mainly macrolide) combination was most pronounced in the more severely ill patients (17.9% mortality vs. 29.7% for fluoroquinolone combinations in patients with PSI category IV or V patients). As fluoroquinolones have equivalent atypical pathogen cove-rage, the most likely explanation is the favorable immunomodulatory properties of macrolides.

These studies provide strong evidence that combination antibiotic therapy with a macrolide is associated with improved outcome from severe CAP. The same benefit is not achieved with fluoroquinolone-based combination therapy, suggesting that the benefit is not a result of coverage of atypical pathogen coinfection and more likely due to immunomodulatory effects of the macrolides. These immunomodulatory effects are also not reproduced by the fluoroquinolones, which may actually have an adverse effect on immune function (Williams et al. 2005). However, all of the studies demonstrating a benefit have been either retrospective or observational trials, leaving open the possibility that factors not included in the multivariate analyses may be the actual cause of the mortality difference. Several editorials have therefore called for a prospective randomized trial of combination macrolide therapy in severe CAP (Waterer 2003, 2005; Weiss et al. 2004). However, a recent randomized control trial in patients with sepsis due to ventilator associated pneumonia treated with clarithromycin did not show a survival benefit (Giamarellos-Bourboulis et al. 2008). On the other hand, clarithromycin accelerated the resolution of ventilator associated pneumonia, and weaning from mechanical ventilation in surviving patients and delayed death in those who died of sepsis.

An even greater issue is whether the benefit of macrolides extends to other infections. A few of the studies included primary or concomitant pneumococcal meningitis or primary bacteremia. However, the benefit in principally gram-negative infections, such as intra-abdominal or urinary tract, is more uncertain. The animal data (Giamarellos-Bourboulis et al. 2005a,b) and the clinical benefit in cystic fibrosis (Kraft et al. 2002; Wolter et al. 2002a,b; Saiman et al. 2003; Gotfried 2004; Kostadima et al. 2004; Schultz 2004; Amsden 2005; Johnston et al. 2006; Piacentini et al. 2007) and bronchiectasis (Koh et al. 1997; Yalcin et al. 2006) do support a clinical trial for gram-negative infections as well. CAP usually accounts for up to 40% of cases of severe sepsis or septic shock in large multicenter therapeutic trials (Bernard et al. 2001) and may even be the major subgroup driving results in the overall trial (Laterre et al. 2005). Concern for the differential benefit in non-CAP infections does warrant stratification of randomization to ensure a balance of CAP patients in each group.

1.7 Conclusion

This chapter summarizes the evidence that macrolide therapy may be useful in the treatment of severe sepsis and severe community-acquired pneumonia. Further randomized clinical trials are needed to clarify the mechanisms why macrolide therapy could modulate the immune response and the impact on clinical outcomes in patients with severe sepsis due to any origin.

The views expressed in this article are those of the authors and do not necessarily represent the views of the Department of Veterans Affairs.

References

Abdelghaffar H, Vazifeh D, and Labro MT (1997) Erythromycin A-derived macrolides modify the functional activities of human neutrophils by altering the phospholipase D-phosphatidate phosphohydrolase transduction pathway L-cladinose is involved both in alterations of neutrophil functions and modulation of this transductional pathway. J Immunol 159:3995–4005.

Abraham E, Wunderink R, Silverman H, Perl TM, Nasraway S, Levy H, et al. (1995) Efficacy and safety of monoclonal antibody to human tumor necrosis factor alpha in patients with sepsis syndrome. A randomized, controlled, double-blind, multicenter clinical trial. TNF-alpha MAb Sepsis Study Group. JAMA 273:934–941.

Abraham E, Anzueto A, Gutierrez G, Tessler S, San Pedro G, Wunderink R, et al. (1998) Double-blind randomised controlled trial of monoclonal antibody to human tumour necrosis factor in treatment of septic shock. NORASEPT II Study Group. Lancet 351:929–933.

Abraham E, Glauser MP, Butler T, Garbino J, Gelmont D, Laterre PF, et al. (1997) p55 Tumor necrosis factor receptor fusion protein in the treatment of patients with severe sepsis and septic shock. A randomized controlled multicenter trial. Ro 45–2081 Study Group. JAMA 277:1531–1538.

Abraham E, Laterre PF, Garbino J, Pingleton S, Butler T, Dugernier T, et al. (2001) Lenercept (p55 tumor necrosis factor receptor fusion protein) in severe sepsis and early septic shock: a randomized, double-blind, placebo-controlled, multicenter phase III trial with 1,342 patients. Crit Care Med 29:503–510.

Abraham E, Laterre PF, Garg R, Levy H, Talwar D, Trzaskoma BL, et al. (2005) Drotrecogin alfa (activated) for adults with severe sepsis and a low risk of death. N Engl J Med 353:1332–1341.

Amayasu H, Yoshida S, Ebana S, Yamamoto Y, Nishikawa T, Shoji T, et al. (2000) Clarithromycin suppresses bronchial hyperresponsiveness associated with eosinophilic inflammation in patients with asthma. Ann Allergy Asthma Immunol 84:594–598.

Amsden GW (2005) Anti-inflammatory effects of macrolides – an underappreciated benefit in the treatment of community-acquired respiratory tract infections and chronic inflammatory pulmonary conditions? J Antimicrob Chemother 55:10–21.

Angus DC, Linde-Zwirble WT, Lidicker J, Clermont G, Carcillo J, and Pinsky MR (2001) Epidemiology of severe sepsis in the United States: analysis of incidence, outcome, and associated costs of care. Crit Care Med 29:1303–1310.

Annane D, Sebille V, Charpentier C, Bollaert PE, Francois B, Korach JM, et al. (2002) Effect of treatment with low doses of hydrocortisone and fludrocortisone on mortality in patients with septic shock. JAMA 288:862–871.

Annane D, Bellissant E, and Cavaillon JM (2005) Septic shock. Lancet 365:63–78.

Austrian R and Gold J (1964) Pneumococcal bacteremia with special reference to bacteremic pneumococcal pneumonia. Ann Intern Med 60:759–776.

Baddour LM, Yu VL, Klugman KP, Feldman C, Ortqvist A, Rello J, et al. (2004) Combination antibiotic therapy lowers mortality among severely ill patients with pneumococcal bacteremia. Am J Respir Crit Care Med 170:440–444.

Basyigit I, Yildiz F, Ozkara SK, Yildirim E, Boyaci H, and Ilgazli A (2004) The effect of clarithromycin on inflammatory markers in chronic obstructive pulmonary disease: preliminary data. Ann Pharmacother 38:1400–1405.

Beringer P, Huynh KM, Kriengkauykiat J, Bi L, Hoem N, Louie S, et al. (2005) Absolute bioavailability and intracellular pharmacokinetics of azithromycin in patients with cystic fibrosis. Antimicrob Agents Chemother 49:5013–5017.

Bernard GR, Vincent JL, Laterre PF, LaRosa SP, Dhainaut JF, Lopez-Rodriguez A, et al. (2001) Efficacy and safety of recombinant human activated protein C for severe sepsis. N Engl J Med 344:699–709.

Beutler B (1993) Endotoxin, tumor necrosis factor, and related mediators: new approaches to shock. New Horiz 1:3–12.

Beutler B, Milsark IW, and Cerami AC (1985) Passive immunization against cachectin/tumor necrosis factor protects mice from lethal effect of endotoxin. Science 229:869–871.

Bone RC (1996) Why sepsis trials fail. JAMA 276:565–566.

Brown RB, Iannini P, Gross P, and Kunkel M (2003) Impact of initial antibiotic choice on clinical outcomes in community-acquired pneumonia: analysis of a hospital claims-made database. Chest 123:1503–1511.

Carlson DL, Willis MS, White DJ, Horton JW, and Giroir BP (2005) Tumor necrosis factor-alpha-induced caspase activation mediates endotoxin-related cardiac dysfunction. Crit Care Med 33:1021–1028.

Casey LC, Balk RA, and Bone RC (1993) Plasma cytokine and endotoxin levels correlate with survival in patients with the sepsis syndrome. Ann Intern Med 119:771–778.

Chow LW, Yuen KY, Woo PC, and Wei WI (2000) Clarithromycin attenuates mastectomy-induced acute inflammatory response. Clin Diagn Lab Immunol 7:925–931.

Clement A, Tamalet A, Leroux E, Ravilly S, Fauroux B, and Jais JP (2006) Long term effects of azithromycin in patients with cystic fibrosis: a double blind, placebo controlled trial. Thorax 61:895–902.

Cohen J and Carlet J (1996) INTERSEPT: an international, multicenter, placebo-controlled trial of monoclonal antibody to human tumor necrosis factor-alpha in patients with sepsis. International Sepsis Trial Study Group. Crit Care Med 24:1431–1440.

Creaven PJ, Brenner DE, Cowens JW, Huben RP, Wolf RM, Takita H, et al. (1989) A phase I clinical trial of recombinant human tumor necrosis factor given daily for five days. Cancer Chemother Pharmacol 23:186–191.

Culic O, Erakovic V, Cepelak I, Barisic K, Brajsa K, Ferencic Z, et al. (2002) Azithromycin modulates neutrophil function and circulating inflammatory mediators in healthy human subjects. Eur J Pharmacol 450:277–289.

Dalhoff A and Shalit I (2003) Immunomodulatory effects of quinolones. Lancet Infect Dis 3:359–371.

Deans KJ, Haley M, Natanson C, Eichacker PQ, and Minneci PC (2005) Novel therapies for sepsis: a review. J Trauma-Inj Infect Crit Care 58:867–874.

Debets JM, Kampmeijer R, van der Linden MP, Buurman WA, and van der Linden CJ (1989) Plasma tumor necrosis factor and mortality in critically ill septic patients. Crit Care Med 17:489–494.

Desaki M, Takizawa H, Ohtoshi T, Kasama T, Kobayashi K, Sunazuka T, et al. (2000) Erythromycin suppresses nuclear factor-kappa B and activator protein-1 activation in human bronchial epithelial cells. Biochem Biophys Res Commun 267:124–128.

Dofferhoff AS, Bom VJ, de Vries-Hospers HG, van Ingen J, vd Meer J, Hazenberg BP, et al. (1992) Patterns of cytokines, plasma endotoxin, plasminogen activator inhibitor, and acute-phase proteins during the treatment of severe sepsis in humans. Crit Care Med 20:185–192.

Dudas V, Hopefl A, Jacobs R, and Guglielmo BJ (2000) Antimicrobial selection for hospitalized patients with presumed community-acquired pneumonia: a survey of nonteaching US community hospitals. Ann Pharmacother 34:446–452.

Eichacker PQ, Parent C, Kalil A, Esposito C, Cui X, Banks SM, et al. (2002) Risk and the efficacy of antiinflammatory agents: retrospective and confirmatory studies of sepsis. Am J Respir Crit Care Med 166:1197–1205.

Eichacker PQ, Danner RL, Suffredini AF, Cui X, and Natanson C (2005) Reassessing recombinant human activated protein C for sepsis: time for a new randomized controlled trial. Crit Care Med 33:2426–2428.

Eichenholz PW, Eichacker PQ, Hoffman WD, Banks SM, Parrillo JE, Danner RL, et al. (1992) Tumor necrosis factor challenges in canines: patterns of cardiovascular dysfunction. Am J Physiol 263:H668–H675.

Equi A, Balfour-Lynn IM, Bush A, and Rosenthal M (2002) Long term azithromycin in children with cystic fibrosis: a randomised, placebo-controlled crossover trial. Lancet 360:978–984.

Ferguson NR, Galley HF, and Webster NR (1999) T helper cell subset ratios in patients with severe sepsis. Intensive Care Med 25:106–109.

Fisher CJ, Jr., Agosti JM, Opal SM, Lowry SF, Balk RA, Sadoff JC, et al. (1996) Treatment of septic shock with the tumor necrosis factor receptor:Fc fusion protein. The Soluble TNF Receptor Sepsis Study Group. N Engl J Med 334:1697–1702.

Fumeaux T, Dufour J, Stern S, and Pugin J (2004) Immune monitoring of patients with septic shock by measurement of intraleukocyte cytokines. Intensive Care Med 30:2028–2037.

Garcia Vazquez E, Mensa J, Martinez JA, Marcos MA, Puig J, Ortega M, et al. (2005) Lower mortality among patients with community-acquired pneumonia treated with a macrolide plus a beta-lactam agent versus a beta-lactam agent alone. Eur J Clin Microbiol Infect Dis 24:190–195.

Gerhardt SG, McDyer JF, Girgis RE, Conte JV, Yang SC, and Orens JB (2003) Maintenance azithromycin therapy for bronchiolitis obliterans syndrome: results of a pilot study. Am J Respir Crit Care Med 168:121–125.

Giamarellos-Bourboulis EJ, Adamis T, Laoutaris G, Sabracos L, Koussoulas V, Mouktaroudi M, et al. (2004) Immunomodulatory clarithromycin treatment of experimental sepsis and acute pyelonephritis caused by multidrug-resistant Pseudomonas aeruginosa. Antimicrob Agents Chemother 48:93–99.

Giamarellos-Bourboulis E, Adamis T, Sabracos L, Raftogiannis M, Baziaka F, Tsaganos T, et al. (2005a) Clarithromycin: immunomodulatory therapy of experimental sepsis and acute pyelonephritis by Escherichia coli. Scand J Infect Dis 37:48–54.

Giamarellos-Bourboulis EJ, Baziaka F, Antonopoulou A, Koutoukas P, Kousoulas V, Sabracos L, et al. (2005b) Clarithromycin co-administered with amikacin attenuates systemic inflammation in experimental sepsis with Escherichia coli. Int J Antimicrob Agents 25:168–172.

Giamarellos-Bourboulis EJ, Pechère JC, Routsi C, Plachouras D, Kollias S, Raftogiannis M, et al. (2008) Effect of Clarithromycin in Patients with Sepsis and Ventilator-Associated Pneumonia. Clin Infect Dis 46:1157–1164.

Gotfried MH (2004) Macrolides for the treatment of chronic sinusitis, asthma, and COPD. Chest 125:52S–60S; quiz 60S–61S.

Hall IH, Schwab U, Ward ES, and Ives T (2004) In vitro anti-inflammatory effects and immunomodulation by gemifloxacin in stimulated human THP-1 monocytes. Pharmazie 59:713–719.

Hatipoglu U and Rubinstein I (2004) Low-dose, long-term macrolide therapy in asthma: an overview. Clin Mol Allergy 2:4.

Hendeles L (1992) Erythromycin for the treatment of bronchial hyperresponsiveness in asthma. Chest 101:296.

Hoiby N (2002) New antimicrobials in the management of cystic fibrosis. J Antimicrob Chemother 49:235–238.

Houck PM, MacLehose RF, Niederman MS, and Lowery JK (2001) Empiric antibiotic therapy and mortality among medicare pneumonia inpatients in 10 western states: 1993, 1995, and 1997. Chest 119:1420–1426.

Hoyert DL, Kung HC, and Smith BL (2005) Deaths: preliminary data for 2003. Natl Vital Stat Rep 53:1–48.

Ishiguro M, Koga H, Kohno S, Hayashi T, Yamaguchi K, and Hirota M (1989) Penetration of macrolides into human polymorphonuclear leucocytes. J Antimicrob Chemother 24:719–729.

Johnston SL, Blasi F, Black PN, Martin RJ, Farrell DJ, Nieman RB, et al. (2006) The effect of telithromycin in acute exacerbations of asthma. N Engl J Med 354:1589–1600.

Kadota J, Mukae H, Ishii H, Nagata T, Kaida H, Tomono K, et al. (2003) Long-term efficacy and safety of clarithromycin treatment in patients with diffuse panbronchiolitis. Respir Med 97:844–850.

Kawasaki S, Takizawa H, Ohtoshi T, Takeuchi N, Kohyama T, Nakamura H, et al. (1998) Roxithromycin inhibits cytokine production by and neutrophil attachment to human bronchial epithelial cells in vitro. Antimicrob Agents Chemother 42:1499–1502.

Khair OA, Devalia JL, Abdelaziz MM, Sapsford RJ, and Davies RJ (1995) Effect of erythromycin on Haemophilus influenzae endotoxin-induced release of IL-6, IL-8 and sICAM-1 by cultured human bronchial epithelial cells. Eur Respir J 8:1451–1457.

Khan AA, Slifer TR, Araujo FG, and Remington JS (1999) Effect of clarithromycin and azithromycin on production of cytokines by human monocytes. Int J Antimicrob Agents 11:121–132.

Kikuchi T, Hagiwara K, Honda Y, Gomi K, Kobayashi T, Takahashi H, et al. (2002) Clarithromycin suppresses lipopolysaccharide-induced interleukin-8 production by human monocytes through AP-1 and NF-kappa B transcription factors. J Antimicrob Chemother 49:745–755.

Kobayashi M, Shimauchi T, Hino R, and Tokura Y (2004) Roxithromycin downmodulates Th2 chemokine production by keratinocytes and chemokine receptor expression on Th2 cells: its dual inhibitory effects on the ligands and the receptors. Cell Immunol 228:27–33.

Koh YY, Lee MH, Sun YH, Sung KW, and Chae JH (1997) Effect of roxithromycin on airway responsiveness in children with bronchiectasis: a double-blind, placebo-controlled study. Eur Respir J 10:994–999.

Kohri K, Tamaoki J, Kondo M, Aoshiba K, Tagaya E, and Nagai A (2000) Macrolide antibiotics inhibit nitric oxide generation by rat pulmonary alveolar macrophages. Eur Respir J 15:62–67.

Kostadima E, Tsiodras S, Alexopoulos EI, Kaditis AG, Mavrou I, Georgatou N, et al. (2004) Clarithromycin reduces the severity of bronchial hyperresponsiveness in patients with asthma. Eur Respir J 23:714–717.

Kraft M, Cassell GH, Pak J, and Martin RJ (2002) Mycoplasma pneumoniae and Chlamydia pneumoniae in asthma: effect of clarithromycin. Chest 121:1782–1788.

Kudoh S, Azuma A, Yamamoto M, Izumi T, and Ando M (1998) Improvement of survival in patients with diffuse panbronchiolitis treated with low-dose erythromycin. Am J Respir Crit Care Med 157:1829–1832.

Kuno R, Wang J, Kawanokuchi J, Takeuchi H, Mizuno T, and Suzumura A (2005) Autocrine activation of microglia by tumor necrosis factor-alpha. J Neuroimmunol 162:89–96.

Laterre PF, Garber G, Levy H, Wunderink R, Kinasewitz GT, Sollet JP, et al. (2005) Severe community-acquired pneumonia as a cause of severe sepsis: data from the PROWESS study. Crit Care Med 33:952–961.

Lenk H, Tanneberger S, Muller U, Ebert J, and Shiga T (1989) Phase II clinical trial of high-dose recombinant human tumor necrosis factor. Cancer Chemother Pharmacol 24:391–392.

Mandell LA, Bartlett JG, Dowell SF, File TM, Jr., Musher DM. and Whitney C (2003) Update of practice guidelines for the management of community-acquired pneumonia in immunocompetent adults. Clin Infect Dis 37:1405–1433.

Martin GS, Mannino DM, Eaton S, and Moss M (2003) The epidemiology of sepsis in the United States from 1979 through 2000. N Engl J Med 348:1546–1554.

Martinez JA, Horcajada JP, Almela M, Marco F, Soriano A, Garcia E, et al. (2003) Addition of a macrolide to a beta-lactam-based empirical antibiotic regimen is associated with lower in-hospital mortality for patients with bacteremic pneumococcal pneumonia. Clin Infect Dis 36:389–395.

Michie HR, Manogue KR, Spriggs DR, Revhaug A, O'Dwyer S, Dinarello CA, et al. (1988) Detection of circulating tumor necrosis factor after endotoxin administration. N Engl J Med 318:1481–1486.

Mikamo H, Kawazoe K, Sato Y, and Tamaya T (1998) Effects of long-term/low-dose clarithromycin on neutrophil count and interleukin-8 level in pyometra. Chemotherapy 44:50–54.

Mitsuyama T, Tanaka T, Hidaka K, Abe M, and Hara N (1995) Inhibition by erythromycin of superoxide anion production by human polymorphonuclear leukocytes through the action of cyclic AMP-dependent protein kinase. Respiration 62:269–273.

Miyatake H, Suzuki K, Taki F, Takagi K, and Satake T (1991a) Effect of erythromycin on bronchial hyperresponsiveness in patients with bronchial asthma. Arzneimittelforschung 41:552–556.

Miyatake H, Taki F, Taniguchi H, Suzuki R, Takagi K, and Satake T (1991b) Erythromycin reduces the severity of bronchial hyperresponsiveness in asthma. Chest 99:670–673.

Mortensen E, Restrepo M, Anzueto A, and Pugh J (2006a) The impact of empiric antimicrobial therapy with a beta-lactam and fluoroquinolone on mortality for patients hospitalized with severe pneumonia. Crit Care 10:R8.

Mortensen EM, Restrepo MI, Anzueto A, and Pugh JA (2006b) Antibiotic therapy and 48-hour mortality for patients with pneumonia. Am J Med 119:859–864.

Mufson MA and Stanek RJ (1999) Bacteremic pneumococcal pneumonia in one American city: a 20-year longitudinal study, 1978–1997. Am J Med 107:34S–43S.

Oishi K, Sonoda F, Kobayashi S, Iwagaki A, Nagatake T, Matsushima K, et al. (1994) Role of interleukin-8 (IL-8) and an inhibitory effect of erythromycin on IL-8 release in the airways of patients with chronic airway diseases. Infect Immun 62:4145–4152.

Panacek EA, Marshall JC, Albertson TE, Johnson DH, Johnson S, MacArthur RD, et al. (2004) Efficacy and safety of the monoclonal anti-tumor necrosis factor antibody F(ab')2 fragment afelimomab in patients with severe sepsis and elevated interleukin-6 levels. Crit Care Med 32:2173–2182.

Parnham MJ, Culic O, Erakovic V, Munic V, Popovic-Grle S, Barisic K, et al. (2005) Modulation of neutrophil and inflammation markers in chronic obstructive pulmonary disease by short-term azithromycin treatment. Eur J Pharmacol 517:132–143.

Parrillo J.E, Parker MM, Natanson C, Suffredini AF, Danner RL, Cunnion RE, et al. (1990) Septic shock in humans. Advances in the understanding of pathogenesis, cardiovascular dysfunction, and therapy. Ann Intern Med 113:227–242.

Piacentini GL, Peroni DG, Bodini A, Pigozzi R, Costella S, Loiacono A, et al. (2007) Azithromycin reduces bronchial hyperresponsiveness and neutrophilic airway inflammation in asthmatic children: a preliminary report. Allergy Asthma Proc 28:194–198.

Rangel-Frausto MS, Pittet D, Costigan M, Hwang T, Davis CS, and Wenzel RP (1995) The natural history of the systemic inflammatory response syndrome (SIRS). A prospective study. JAMA 273:117–123.

Reinhart K, Wiegand-Lohnert C, Grimminger F, Kaul M, Withington S, Treacher D, et al. (1996) Assessment of the safety and efficacy of the monoclonal anti-tumor necrosis factor antibody-fragment, MAK 195F, in patients with sepsis and septic shock: a multicenter, randomized, placebo-controlled, dose-ranging study. Crit Care Med 24:733–742.

Reinhart K and Karzai W (2001) Anti-tumor necrosis factor therapy in sepsis: update on clinical trials and lessons learned. Crit Care Med 29:S121–S125.

Rodríguez A, Mendia A, Sirvent JM, Barcenilla F, de la Torre-Prados MV, Solé-Violán J, Rello J; CAPUCI Study Group. (2007) Combination antibiotic therapy improves survival in patients with community-acquired pneumonia and shock. Crit Care Med 35:1493–1498.

Rodvold KA (1999) Clinical pharmacokinetics of clarithromycin. Clin Pharmacokinet 37:385–398.

Ruiz M, Ewig S, Torres A, Arancibia F, Marco F, Mensa J, et al. (1999) Severe community-acquired pneumonia. Risk factors and follow-up epidemiology. Am J Respir Crit Care Med 160:923–929.

Saiman L, Marshall BC, Mayer-Hamblett N, Burns JL, Quittner AL, Cibene DA, et al. (2003) Azithromycin in patients with cystic fibrosis chronically infected with Pseudomonas aeruginosa: a randomized controlled trial. JAMA 290:1749–1756.

Schultz MJ, Speelman P, Hack CE, Buurman WA, van Deventer SJH, and van der Poll T (2000) Intravenous infusion of erythromycin inhibits CXC chemokine production, but augments neutrophil degranulation in whole blood stimulated with Streptococcus pneumoniae. J Antimicrob Chemother 46:235–240.

Schultz MJ (2004) Macrolide activities beyond their antimicrobial effects: macrolides in diffuse panbronchiolitis and cystic fibrosis. J Antimicrob Chemother 54:21–28.

Southern KW and Barker PM (2004) Azithromycin for cystic fibrosis. Eur Respir J 24:834–838.

Stover DE and Mangino D (2005) Macrolides: a treatment alternative for bronchiolitis obliterans organizing pneumonia? Chest 128:3611–3617.

Tamaoki J (2004) The effects of macrolides on inflammatory cells. Chest 125:41S–50S; quiz 51S.

Tamaoki J, Kadota J, and Takizawa H (2004) Clinical implications of the immunomodulatory effects of macrolides. Am J Med 117(Suppl 9A):5S–11S.

Tracey KJ, Fong Y, Hesse DG, Manogue KR, Lee AT, Kuo GC, et al. (1987) Anti-cachectin/TNF monoclonal antibodies prevent septic shock during lethal bacteraemia. Nature 330:662–664.

Van Amersfoort ES, Van Berkel TJ, and Kuiper J (2003) Receptors, mediators, and mechanisms involved in bacterial sepsis and septic shock. Clin Microbiol Rev 16:379–414.

van Leeuwen HJ, Van Der Tol M, Van Strijp JA, Verhoef J, and van Kessel KP (2005) The role of tumour necrosis factor in the kinetics of lipopolysaccharide-mediated neutrophil priming in whole blood. Clin Exp Immunol 140:65–72.

Vazifeh D, Bryskier A, and Labro MT (2000) Effect of proinflammatory cytokines on the interplay between roxithromycin, HMR 3647, or HMR 3004 and human polymorphonuclear neutrophils. Antimicrob Agents Chemother 44:511–521.

Verleden GM, Vanaudenaerde BM, Dupont LJ, and Van Raemdonck DE (2006) Azithromycin reduces airway neutrophilia and interleukin-8 in patients with bronchiolitis obliterans syndrome. Am J Respir Crit Care Med 174:566–570.

Vila-del Sol V and Fresno M (2005) Involvement of TNF and NF-kappa B in the transcriptional control of cyclooxygenase-2 expression by IFN-gamma in macrophages. J Immunol 174:2825–2833.

Vincent JL, de Mendonca A, Cantraine F, Moreno R, Takala J, Suter PM, et al. (1998) Use of the SOFA score to assess the incidence of organ dysfunction/failure in intensive care units: results of a multicenter, prospective study. Working group on "sepsis-related problems" of the European Society of Intensive Care Medicine. Crit Care Med 26:1793–1800.

Waterer GW (2003) Combination antibiotic therapy with macrolides in community-acquired pneumonia: more smoke but is there any fire? Chest 123:1328–1329.

Waterer GW (2005) Optimal antibiotic treatment in severe pneumococcal pneumonia - time for real answers. Eur J Clin Microbiol Infect Dis 24:691–692.

Waterer GW, Somes GW, and Wunderink RG (2001) Monotherapy may be suboptimal for severe bacteremic pneumococcal pneumonia. Arch Intern Med 161:1837–1842.

Weiss K, Low DE, Cortes L, Beaupre A, Gauthier R, Gregoire P, et al. (2004) Clinical characteristics at initial presentation and impact of dual therapy on the outcome of bacteremic Streptococcus pneumoniae pneumonia in adults. Can Respir J 11:589–593.

Williams AC, Galley HF, Watt AM, and Webster NR (2005) Differential effects of three antibiotics on T helper cell cytokine expression. J Antimicrob Chemother 56:502–506.

Wolter J, Seeney S, Bell S, Bowler S, Masel P, and McCormack J (2002a) Effect of long term treatment with azithromycin on disease parameters in cystic fibrosis: a randomised trial. Thorax 57:212–216.

Wolter JM, Seeney SL, and McCormack JG (2002b) Macrolides in cystic fibrosis: is there a role? Am J Respir Med 1:235–241.

Yalcin E, Kiper N, Ozcelik U, Dogru D, Firat P, Sahin A, et al. (2006) Effects of clarithromycin on inflammatory parameters and clinical conditions in children with bronchiectasis. J Clin Pharm Ther 31:49–55.

Yamamoto M, Kondo A, Tamura M, Izumi T, Ina Y, and Noda M (1990) Long-term therapeutic effects of erythromycin and newquinolone antibacterial agents on diffuse panbronchiolitis. Nihon Kyobu Shikkan Gakkai Zasshi 28:1305–1313.

Yamanaka Y, Tamari M, Nakahata T, and Nakamura Y (2001) Gene expression profiles of human small airway epithelial cells treated with low doses of 14- and 16-membered macrolides. Biochem Biophys Res Commun 287:198–203.

Zeni F, Freeman B, and Natanson C (1997) Anti-inflammatory therapies to treat sepsis and septic shock: a reassessment. Crit Care Med 25:1095–1100.

Chapter 2
The Potential Role of Statins in Severe Sepsis

Eric M. Mortensen, Marcos I. Restrepo, and Antonio Anzueto

2.1 Introduction

Sepsis is the tenth leading cause of death in the United States (Hoyert et al. 2001) and has a mortality rate of up to 70% (Angus et al. 2001; Annane et al. 2003). Inpatients with sepsis have a 26-fold increased risk of death compared to intensive care unit subjects without sepsis (Annane et al. 2003). New medications are urgently needed to prevent and treat sepsis since only a few new classes of antibiotics have been added to the armamentarium in the past ten years, and only one new class of medication specifically targeting sepsis (drotrecogin-alfa) has been added (Bernard et al. 2001).

In the United States, almost $17 billion is spent each year treating patients with sepsis (Angus et al. 2001). More than 750,000 cases of severe sepsis occur annually (Angus et al. 2001), with the incidence increasing due to the aging population, the growing number of immunocompromised patients, increasing use of invasive procedures, and increasing antibiotic resistance. Despite advances in care, the mortality rate due to severe sepsis remains up to 80% (Annane et al. 2003). Even single organ dysfunction is associated with a mortality rate of 20% with mortality increasing by up to 20% for each additional dysfunctional organ (Vincent et al. 1998).

Recently, several classes of medications including HMG-CoA reductase inhibitors (statins) have been found to attenuate the systemic inflammatory response (de Bont et al. 1998; Jialal et al. 2001; Musial et al. 2001; Ridker et al. 1998; Rosenson and Tangney 1998; Rosenson et al. 1999; Strandberg et al. 1999). In addition, statins have been demonstrated to have protective endothelial effects, influence inflammatory cell signaling, directly effect T-cell activity, and influence the nitric oxide balance to promote hemodynamic stability (Almog 2003; Hothersall et al. 2006; Terblanche et al. 2007). Several epidemiologic studies have demonstrated that subjects receiving statins hospitalized with bacteremia and community-acquired pneumonia have improved clinical outcomes, or decreased incidence of sepsis (Almog et al. 2004, 2007; Fernandez et al. 2006; Frost et al. 2007; Gupta et al. 2007; Hackam et al. 2006; Kruger et al. 2006; Liappis et al. 2001; Martin et al. 2007; Mortensen et al. 2005a,b; Schlienger et al. 2007; Thomsen et al. 2006; Yang et al. 2007).

The purpose of this article is to review the scientific literature regarding the potential role of statins in the prevention and/or treatment of severe sepsis.

J. Rello, M.I. Restrepo (eds.) *Sepsis: New Strategies for Management.*
doi:10.1007/978-3-540-79001-3 © Springer-Verlag 2008

2.2 Statins

A growing body of evidence suggests that the magnitude of effect of statins on cardiovascular outcomes may be greater than their attributable effect on lowering cholesterol (Arntz 1999; Koenig 2000). This evidence suggests that a secondary
mechanism of action may include increasing inflammatory responses that are either
primary or secondary contributors to progression of atherosclerosis, which is similar
to the pathogenesis of sepsis (Ross 1999). Inflammation is considered the first line
of defense in host–pathogen interactions. The inflammatory process is necessary so
that pathogens are contained and eliminated, and the ability of an organism to mount
and successfully resolve inflammatory responses is imperative to the subsequent
health of that organism (Cazzola et al. 2005). Inflammation is mediated by a
number of cytokines including proinflammatory cytokines such as interleukin (IL)-
1, IL-6, and tumor necrosis factor (TNF)-a; and anti-inflammatory cytokines such
as IL-10 and transforming growth factor (TGF)-b. These cytokines are necessary
for proper function of the immune system, but the overexpression, or inappropriate
expression of these proinflammatory cytokines can result in tissue destruction, sepsis, or death (Nathan 2002). At least four studies have documented short-term
(7 week to 12 month) declines in one or more of the following cytokines/inflamma-
tory markers after treatment with statins: C-reactive protein, TNF-α, or IL-6 in
patients taking statins for hypercholesterolemia (Jialal et al. 2001; Musial et al.
2001; Rosenson et al. 1999; Weis et al. 2001).

In addition, there are several other potential pathways that statins may exert
effects on the body (Table 2.1). These include effects on T-cell activity, coagulation
and fibrinolysis, antioxidant effects, nitric oxide balance, leukocyte–endothelium
interactions, and inflammatory cell signaling and gene expression (Hothersall et al.

Table 2.1 Physiologic actions of statins

Actions	References
Antioxidant effects	Aviram et al. 1998; Girona et al. 1999; Grosser et al. 2004; Landmesser et al. 2005; Rikitake et al. 2001; Shishehbor et al. 2003; Yamamoto et al. 1998
Coagulation	Bickel et al. 2002; Bourcier et al. 2000; Shi et al. 2003; Steiner et al. 2005
Cellular apoptosis	Hakamada-Taguchi et al. 2003; Newton et al. 2002; Rudich et al. 1998
Cytokine release	Ando et al. 2000; Diomede et al. 2001; Ikeda and Shimada 1999; Ikeda et al. 1999; Kleemann et al. 2004; Nath et al. 2004; Steiner et al. 2005; Wang et al. 2005
Inflammatory cell signaling	Dichtl et al. 2003; Grip et al. 2002; Jacobson et al. 2005; Kleemann et al. 2004
Leukocyte–endothelial cell adhesion	Diomede et al. 2001; Grip et al. 2002; Jacobson et al. 2005; Kallen et al. 1999; Kimura et al. 1997; Kothe et al. 2000; Lefer et al. 2001; Ni et al. 2001; Pruefer et al. 2002; Rice et al. 2003; Romano et al. 2000; Scalia et al. 2001; Yoshida et al. 2001
Nitric oxide balance	Grosser et al. 2004; Landmesser et al. 2005

2006; Terblanche et al. 2007). These so-called pleiotropic effects of statins have numerous potential sites of action, and it is unclear which potential mechanisms for the observational studies demonstrate a protective association between statin use and infectious diseases.

There are several potential adverse effects for statins in sepsis that should be acknowledged. Besides previously demonstrated adverse effects of statins such as rhabdomyolysis and hepatotoxocity, other studies had demonstrated that lipoproteins may be protective against endotoxins so that lowering the serum levels of lipoproteins may be detrimental (Almog 2003; Bonville et al. 2004; Harris et al. 2000). In addition, lower levels of serum cholesterol have been shown to be a predictor of higher hospital mortality and increased risk of various infections, including HIV (Claxton et al. 1998; Iribarren et al. 1998).

2.3 Observational Studies

Several published studies have examined the effect of statin use on infectious disease-related outcomes (Table 2.2). The first published paper by Liappis et al. (2001) studied 388 patients hospitalized with bacteremia, and found a protective effect of in-hospital statin use on in-hospital mortality (6% vs. 28%, $p < 0.002$). After adjusting for confounding factors (including comorbid conditions, age, concurrent medications, site of infection, vital signs, and laboratory data), not being on a statin (odds ratio (OR) 7.6, 95% confidence interval (CI) 1.01–57.5) was associated with increased mortality.

2.3.1 Studies of Sepsis

There have been four published studies that examine the association of statin use on the incidence of sepsis or survival after sepsis. Almog et al. described a prospective study of 361 patients hospitalized with cellulitis, CAP, or urinary tract infections which demonstrated a decreased rate of sepsis for patients who were taking statins versus those who were not (2.4% vs. 19%, $p < 0.001$) (Almog et al. 2004). However, no significant difference was seen in 28-day mortality. Another study recently published in the Lancet describes the results of a population-based cohort study ($n = 141,487$) that examined the impact of statin use to prevent sepsis using administrative databases from Ontario, Canada (Hackam et al. 2006). After adjusting for potential confounders, the incidence of sepsis was lower in patients receiving statins as compared to controls (hazard ratio 0.8, 95% CI 0.7–0.9). However, this paper did not examine the effect of statin use on patients already hospitalized with sepsis. Finally, another recent study was published in JAMA by Gupta et al. (2007) with the aim of examining whether statin use was associated with decreased incidence of hospitalization for sepsis. This prospective cohort study included

Table 2.2 Observational studies of statin use and infectious/pulmonary diseases

Reference	Year	Design	Subjects	Infectious disease	Results
Liappis (Liappis et al. 2001)	2001	Single center, retrospective cohort	388 total 35 on statins	Bacteremia	Increased mortality for those not on statins (OR 7.6, 95% CI 1.01–57)
Almog (Almog et al. 2004)	2004	Single center, prospective cohort	361 total 82 on statins	Severe sepsis incidence	Statins protective against sepsis 2.4% vs. 19%, $p < 0.001$
Mortensen (Mortensen et al. 2005a)	2005	Multicenter, retrospective cohort	787 total 110 on statins	Community-acquired pneumonia	Statins protective (OR 0.36, 95% CI 0.14–0.92)
Fernandez (Fernandez et al. 2006)	2005	Single center, retrospective cohort	438 total, 38 on statins	Mechanically ventilated >96 h, ICU-acquired infections	No difference in infections (29 vs. 38%) and higher mortality for statins (61% vs. 42%
Hackam (Hackam et al. 2006)	2006	Population-based, retrospective cohort	69,168 total 34,584 on statins	Incidence of sepsis per 10,000 person years	71.2 for statins vs. 88 for non-statins ($p = 0.0003$)
Kruger (Kruger et al. 2006)	2006	Single center, retrospective cohort	438 total, 66 on statins	Bacteremia	Mortality less for statins (10.6% vs. 23.1%, $p = 0.02$)
Thomsen (Thomsen et al. 2006)	2006	Population-based, retrospective cohort	5,353 total, 176 on statins	Bacteremia	No difference in 30-day mortality 31–180 mortality less for statins (8.4% vs. 17.5%, $p < 0.05$)
Majumdar (Majumdar et al. 2006)	2006	Multicenter prospective cohort	3,415 total 325 on statins	Community-acquired pneumonia	No difference for in-hospital mortality (8% for statins vs. 10%, $p = 0.2$)
Martin (Martin et al. 2007)	2007	Single center, retrospective cohort	53 total 16 on statins	Incidence of severe sepsis	56% for statins group vs. 86%, $p < 0.02$
Yang (Yang et al. 2007)	2007	Single center, retrospective cohort	454 total 104 statins	Sepsis	No difference in 30-day mortality with statin use (19.2% vs. 18.9%, $p = 0.95$)
Schlienger (Schlienger et al. 2007)	2007	Population-based, retrospective case control	1,253 pneumonia cases 4,838 controls	Incidence of pneumonia	Statin users had reduced risk of fatal pneumonia (OR 0.47, 95% CI 0.25–0.88)
Gupta (Gupta et al. 2007)	2007	Multicenter, prospective cohort study	1,041 total 143 statins	Incidence of sepsis	Statin use protective against sepsis (incident rate ratio 0.24, 95% CI 0.11–0.49)
Almog (Almog et al. 2007)	2007	Single center, prospective cohort	11,362 total 5,698 statins	Infection-related mortality	Statins users had significantly lower mortality (hazard ratio 0.37, 95% CI 0.27–0.52)
Frost (Frost et al. 2007)	2007	Population-based, retrospective cohort and case control	76,232 total 11,583 statins	Mortality due to influenza/pneumonia	Statin use associated with decreased mortality (OR 0.6, 95% CI 0.44– 0.81)

1,041 incident dialysis patients at 81 centers and followed them for a mean of 3.4 years. They found that, after adjustment for potential confounders using propensity matching, statin use was strongly protective against sepsis (OR 0.24, 95% CI 0.11–0.49).

The only study of statins and sepsis not to find a potentially protective association was recently published in the *American Journal of Emergency Medicine*. Yang et al. (2007) examined 454 Taiwanese subjects hospitalized with sepsis. After adjusting for potential confounders, they found no significant difference in 30-day mortality (risk ratio 0.95, 95% CI 0.53–1.68). There was a trend toward lower mortality in those with gram-negative sepsis (10.3% vs. 16.4%, $p = 0.25$). Unfortunately, since the final models were not presented in the paper, it is unclear, however, how complete the risk adjustment was.

2.3.2 Studies of Pneumonia

There have been several studies of statin use and pneumonia-related outcomes. The first by Mortensen et al. (2005a) was a retrospective cohort study of 787 subjects hospitalized with CAP at two academic tertiary care hospitals to assess the effects of current outpatient statin use on 30-day mortality. Of the 787 subjects, 110 subjects (14%) were on statins, and after adjusting for potential confounders, including severity of illness, the use of statins (OR 0.4, 95% CI 0.1–0.9) was significantly associated with decreased 30-day mortality. Another study by Majumdar et al. (2006) showed no significant difference in mortality for patients with pneumonia who were statin users after adjusting for potential confounders. Although this study had a prospectively derived cohort of 3,415 subjects, there were several problems with this study including an inappropriate composite outcome, unclear model building, and a cohort with significantly lower rates of statin use in key populations as compared to other published studies of statins association with sepsis and/or pneumonia (Mortensen et al. 2006). Another paper by Schlienger et al. described a case-control study of 1,254 pneumonia cases that were matched with 4,838 control patients from a population-based database of 134,262 patients more than 30 years of age (Schlienger et al. 2007). They found that current statin use, but not past use, was associated with reduction in fatal pneumonia (OR 0.47, 95% CI 0.25–0.88).

2.3.3 Studies of Other Infectious and Pulmonary Diseases

In addition to the study by Liappis et al. discussed above, there have been several other studies which examine statins impact on outcomes for other infectious and pulmonary diseases. A retrospective study of 438 patients hospitalized with bacteremia demonstrated a significant difference for in-hospital mortality: 1.8% for patients on statins versus 23.1% for non-statin users ($p = 0.0002$) (Kruger et al. 2006).

Unfortunately, this study had significant limitations including not controlling comorbid conditions or other medications in the multivariable analyses. Another recent prospective population-based study by Almog et al. (2007) of 11,490 patients with cardiovascular disease that were followed by up to 3 years demonstrated that statin use was associated with significantly lower mortality (0.9% vs. 4.1%). A paper by Frost et al. (2007), which presents several analyses including a cohort study and several case-control analyses, found that statin use was associated with decreased odds of influenza/pneumonia death (OR 0.60, 95% CI 0.44–0.81) and COPD death (OR 0.17, 95% CI 0.07–0.42).

In contrast, Fernandez et al. examined 438 ICU patients that were mechanically ventilated for $>96\,$h and demonstrated increased mortality (61% vs. 42%, $p = 0.03$) for those patients who were taking a statin prior to admission (Fernandez et al. 2006). However, this study included only highly selected patients who received at least 4 days of mechanical ventilation prior to inclusion. Therefore this study excluded patients who may have had improved outcomes due to statin use and did not need this duration of mechanical ventilation.

2.4   Conclusion

This chapter summarizes the evidence that statins may be useful in the prevention and/or treatment of severe sepsis. These results add an additional potential benefit of statins to their demonstrated benefits for subjects with vascular and renal disease. Additional research, especially randomized clinical trials, is needed to elucidate whether statins may have a role in prevention of sepsis or treatment of patients hospitalized with severe sepsis.

References

Almog, Y. (2003). Statins, inflammation, and sepsis: Hypothesis. Chest, 124, 740–743.

Almog, Y., Shefer, A., Novack, V., Maimon, N., Barski, L., Eizinger, M., Friger, M., Zeller, L., and Danon, A. (2004). Prior statin therapy is associated with a decreased rate of severe sepsis. Circulation, 110, 880–885.

Almog, Y., Novack, V., Eisinger, M., Porath, A., Novack, L., and Gilutz, H. (2007). The effect of statin therapy on infection-related mortality in patients with atherosclerotic diseases. Crit Care Med, 35, 372–378.

Ando, H., Takamura, T., Ota, T., Nagai, Y., and Kobayashi, K. (2000). Cerivastatin improves survival of mice with lipopolysaccharide-induced sepsis. J Pharmacol Exp Ther, 294, 1043–1046.

Angus, D.C., Linde-Zwirble, W.T., Lidicker, J., Clermont, G., Carcillo, J., and Pinsky, M.R. (2001a). Epidemiology of severe sepsis in the United States: Analysis of incidence, outcome, and associated costs of care. Crit Care Med, 29, 1303–1310.

Annane, D., Aegerter, P., Jars-Guincestre, M.C., and Guidet, B. (2003). Current epidemiology of septic shock: The CUB-Rea network. Am J Respir Crit Care Med, 168, 165–172.

Arntz, H.R. (1999). Evidence for the benefit of early intervention with pravastatin for secondary prevention of cardiovascular events. Atherosclerosis, 147 Suppl 1, S17–S21.

Aviram, M., Rosenblat, M., Bisgaier, C.L., and Newton, R.S. (1998). Atorvastatin and gemfibrozil metabolites, but not the parent drugs, are potent antioxidants against lipoprotein oxidation. Atherosclerosis, 138, 271–280.

Bernard, G.R., Vincent, J.L., Laterre, P.F., LaRosa, S.P., Dhainaut, J.F., Lopez-Rodriguez, A., Steingrub, J.S., Garber, G.E., Helterbrand, J.D., Ely, E.W., and Fisher, C.J., Jr. (2001). Efficacy and safety of recombinant human activated protein C for severe sepsis. N Engl J Med, 344, 699–709.

Bickel, C., Rupprecht, H.J., Blankenberg, S., Espinola-Klein, C., Rippin, G., Hafner, G., Lotz, J., Prellwitz, W., and Meyer, J. (2002). Influence of HMG-CoA reductase inhibitors on markers of coagulation, systemic inflammation and soluble cell adhesion. Int J Cardiol, 82, 25–31.

Bonville, D.A., Parker, T.S., Levine, D.M., Gordon, B.R., Hydo, L.J., Eachempati, S.R., and Barie, P.S. (2004). The relationships of hypocholesterolemia to cytokine concentrations and mortality in critically ill patients with systemic inflammatory response syndrome. Surg Infect (Larchmt), 5, 39–49.

Bourcier, T., and Libby, P. (2000). HMG-CoA reductase inhibitors reduce plasminogen activator inhibitor-1 expression by human vascular smooth muscle and endothelial cells. Arterioscler Thromb Vasc Biol, 20, 556–562.

Cazzola, M., Matera, M.G., and Pezzuto, G. (2005). Inflammation – A new therapeutic target in pneumonia. Respiration, 72, 117–126.

Claxton, A.J., Jacobs, D.R., Jr., Iribarren, C., Welles, S.L., Sidney, S., and Feingold, K.R. (1998). Association between serum total cholesterol and HIV infection in a high-risk cohort of young men. J Acquir Immune Defic Syndr Hum Retrovirol, 17, 51–57.

de Bont, N., Netea, M.G., Rovers, C., Smilde, T., Demacker, P.N., van der Meer, J.W., and Stalenhoef, A.F. (1998). LPS-induced cytokine production and expression of LPS-receptors by peripheral blood mononuclear cells of patients with familial hypercholesterolemia and the effect of HMG-CoA reductase inhibitors. Atherosclerosis, 139, 147–152.

Dichtl, W., Dulak, J., Frick, M., Alber, H.F., Schwarzacher, S.P., Ares, M.P., Nilsson, J., Pachinger, O., and Weidinger, F. (2003). HMG-CoA reductase inhibitors regulate inflammatory transcription factors in human endothelial and vascular smooth muscle cells. Arterioscler Thromb Vasc Biol, 23, 58–63.

Diomede, L., Albani, D., Sottocorno, M., Donati, M.B., Bianchi, M., Fruscella, P., and Salmona, M. (2001). In vivo anti-inflammatory effect of statins is mediated by nonsterol mevalonate products. Arterioscler Thromb Vasc Biol, 21, 1327–1332.

Fernandez, R., De Pedro, V.J., and Artigas, A. (2006). Statin therapy prior to ICU admission: Protection against infection or a severity marker? Intensive Care Med, 32, 160–164.

Frost, F.J., Petersen, H., Tollestrup, K., and Skipper, B. (2007). Influenza and COPD mortality protection as pleiotropic, dose-dependent effects of statins. Chest, 131, 1006–1012.

Girona, J., La Ville, A.E., Sola, R., Plana, N., and Masana, L. (1999). Simvastatin decreases aldehyde production derived from lipoprotein oxidation. Am J Cardiol, 83, 846–851.

Grip, O., Janciauskiene, S., and Lindgren, S. (2002). Atorvastatin activates PPAR-gamma and attenuates the inflammatory response in human monocytes. Inflamm Res, 51, 58–62.

Grosser, N., Erdmann, K., Hemmerle, A., Berndt, G., Hinkelmann, U., Smith, G., and Schroder, H. (2004). Rosuvastatin upregulates the antioxidant defense protein heme oxygenase-1. Biochem Biophys Res Commun, 325, 871–876.

Gupta, R., Plantinga, L.C., Fink, N.E., Melamed, M.L., Coresh, J., Fox, C.S., Levin, N.W., and Powe, N.R. (2007). Statin use and hospitalization for sepsis in patients with chronic kidney disease. JAMA, 297, 1455–1464.

Hackam, D.G., Mamdani, M., and Redelmeier, D.A. (2006). Statins and sepsis in patients with cardiovascular disease: A population-based cohort analysis. Lancet, 367, 413–418.

Hakamada-Taguchi, R., Uehara, Y., Kuribayashi, K., Numabe, A., Saito, K., Negoro, H., Fujita, T., Toyo-oka, T., and Kato, T. (2003). Inhibition of hydroxymethylglutaryl-coenzyme A reductase reduces Th1 development and promotes Th2 development. Circ Res, 93, 948–956.

Harris, H.W., Gosnell, J.E., and Kumwenda, Z.L. (2000). The lipemia of sepsis: Triglyceride-rich lipoproteins as agents of innate immunity. J Endotoxin Res, 6, 421–430.

Hothersall, E., McSharry, C., and Thomson, N.C. (2006). Potential therapeutic role for statins in respiratory disease. Thorax, 61, 729–734.

Hoyert, D.L., Arias, E., and Smith, B.L. (2001). Deaths: Final data for 1999. Natl Vital Stat Rep, 49, 1–113.

Ikeda, U., and Shimada, K. (1999). Statins and monocytes. Lancet, 353, 2070.

Ikeda, U., Ito, T., and Shimada, K. (1999). Statins and C-reactive protein. Lancet, 353, 1274–1275.

Iribarren, C., Jacobs, D.R., Jr., Sidney, S., Claxton, A.J., and Feingold, K.R. (1998). Cohort study of serum total cholesterol and in-hospital incidence of infectious diseases. Epidemiol Infect, 121, 335–347.

Jacobson, J.R., Barnard, J.W., Grigoryev, D.N., Ma, S.F., Tuder, R.M., and Garcia, J.G. (2005). Simvastatin attenuates vascular leak and inflammation in murine inflammatory lung injury. Am J Physiol Lung Cell Mol Physiol, 288, L1026–L1032.

Jialal, I., Stein, D., Balis, D., Grundy, S.M., Adams-Huet, B., and Devaraj, S. (2001). Effect of hydroxymethyl glutaryl coenzyme A reductase inhibitor therapy on high sensitive C-reactive protein levels. Circulation, 103, 1933–1935.

Kallen, J., Welzenbach, K., Ramage, P., Geyl, D., Kriwacki, R., Legge, G., Cottens, S., Weitz-Schmidt, G., and Hommel, U. (1999). Structural basis for LFA-1 inhibition upon lovastatin binding to the CD11a I-domain. J Mol Biol, 292, 1–9.

Kimura, M., Kurose, I., Russell, J., and Granger, D.N. (1997). Effects of fluvastatin on leukocyte-endothelial cell adhesion in hypercholesterolemic rats. Arterioscler Thromb Vasc Biol, 17, 1521–1526.

Kleemann, R., Verschuren, L., de Rooij, B.J., Lindeman, J., de Maat, M.M., Szalai, A.J., Princen, H.M., and Kooistra, T. (2004). Evidence for anti-inflammatory activity of statins and PPAR alpha activators in human C-reactive protein transgenic mice in vivo and in cultured human hepatocytes in vitro. Blood, 103, 4188–4194.

Koenig, W. (2000). Heart disease and the inflammatory response. BMJ, 321, 187–188.

Kothe, H., Dalhoff, K., Rupp, J., Muller, A., Kreuzer, J., Maass, M., and Katus, H.A. (2000). Hydroxymethylglutaryl coenzyme A reductase inhibitors modify the inflammatory response of human macrophages and endothelial cells infected with chlamydia pneumoniae. Circulation, 101, 1760–1763.

Kruger, P., Fitzsimmons, K., Cook, D., Jones, M., and Nimmo, G. (2006). Statin therapy is associated with fewer deaths in patients with bacteraemia. Intensive Care Med, 32, 75–79.

Landmesser, U., Bahlmann, F., Mueller, M., Spiekermann, S., Kirchhoff, N., Schulz, S., Manes, C., Fischer, D., de Groot, K., Fliser, D., Fauler, G., Marz, W., and Drexler, H. (2005). Simvastatin versus ezetimibe: Pleiotropic and lipid-lowering effects on endothelial function in humans. Circulation, 111, 2356–2363.

Lefer, D.J., Scalia, R., Jones, S.P., Sharp, B.R., Hoffmeyer, M.R., Farvid, A.R., Gibson, M.F., and Lefer, A.M. (2001). HMG-CoA reductase inhibition protects the diabetic myocardium from ischemia-reperfusion injury. FASEB J, 15, 1454–1456.

Liappis, A.P., Kan, V.L., Rochester, C.G., and Simon, G.L. (2001). The effect of statins on mortality in patients with bacteremia. Clin Infect Dis, 33, 1352–1357.

Majumdar, S.R., McAlister, F.A., Eurich, D.T., Padwal, R.S., and Marrie, T.J. (2006). Statins and outcomes in patients admitted to hospital with community acquired pneumonia: Population based prospective cohort study. BMJ, 333, 999.

Martin, C.P., Talbert, R.L., Burgess, D.S., and Peters, J.I. (2007). Effectiveness of statins in reducing the rate of severe sepsis: A retrospective evaluation. Pharmacotherapy, 27, 20–26.

Mortensen, E.M., Restrepo, M., Anzueto, A., and Pugh, J. (2005a). The effect of prior statin use on 30-day mortality for patients hospitalized with community-acquired pneumonia. Respir Res, 6, 82.

Mortensen, E.M., Restrepo, M.I., Copeland, L.A., Pugh, M.J., and Anzueto, A. (2006). Statins and outcomes in patients with pneumonia: Not only healthy user bias. BMJ, 333, 1123–1124.

Musial, J., Undas, A., Gajewski, P., Jankowski, M., Sydor, W., and Szczeklik, A. (2001). Anti-inflammatory effects of simvastatin in subjects with hypercholesterolemia. Int J Cardiol, 77, 247–253.

Nath, N., Giri, S., Prasad, R., Singh, A.K., and Singh, I. (2004). Potential targets of 3-hydroxy-3-methylglutaryl coenzyme A reductase inhibitor for multiple sclerosis therapy. J Immunol, 172, 1273–1286.

Nathan, C. (2002). Points of control in inflammation. Nature, 420, 846.

Newton, C.J., Ran, G., Xie, Y.X., Bilko, D., Burgoyne, C.H., Adams, I., Abidia, A., McCollum, P.T., and Atkin, S.L. (2002). Statin-induced apoptosis of vascular endothelial cells is blocked by dexamethasone. J Endocrinol, 174, 7–16.

Ni, W., Egashira, K., Kataoka, C., Kitamoto, S., Koyanagi, M., Inoue, S., and Takeshita, A. (2001). Antiinflammatory and antiarteriosclerotic actions of HMG-CoA reductase inhibitors in a rat model of chronic inhibition of nitric oxide synthesis. Circ Res, 89, 415–421.

Pruefer, D., Makowski, J., Schnell, M., Buerke, U., Dahm, M., Oelert, H., Sibelius, U., Grandel, U., Grimminger, F., Seeger, W., Meyer, J., Darius, H., and Buerke, M. (2002). Simvastatin inhibits inflammatory properties of staphylococcus aureus alpha-toxin. Circulation, 106, 2104–2110.

Rice, J.B., Stoll, L.L., Li, W.G., Denning, G.M., Weydert, J., Charipar, E., Richenbacher, W.E., Miller, F.J., Jr., and Weintraub, N.L. (2003). Low-level endotoxin induces potent inflammatory activation of human blood vessels: Inhibition by statins. Arterioscler Thromb Vasc Biol, 23, 1576–1582.

Ridker, P.M., Rifai, N., Pfeffer, M.A., Sacks, F.M., Moye, L.A., Goldman, S., Flaker, G.C., and Braunwald, E. (1998). Inflammation, pravastatin, and the risk of coronary events after myocardial infarction in patients with average cholesterol levels. Cholesterol and recurrent events (care) investigators. Circulation, 98, 839–844.

Rikitake, Y., Kawashima, S., Takeshita, S., Yamashita, T., Azumi, H., Yasuhara, M., Nishi, H., Inoue, N., and Yokoyama, M. (2001). Anti-oxidative properties of fluvastatin, an HMG-CoA reductase inhibitor, contribute to prevention of atherosclerosis in cholesterol-fed rabbits. Atherosclerosis, 154, 87–96.

Romano, M., Diomede, L., Sironi, M., Massimiliano, L., Sottocorno, M., Polentarutti, N., Guglielmotti, A., Albani, D., Bruno, A., Fruscella, P., Salmona, M., Vecchi, A., Pinza, M., and Mantovani, A. (2000). Inhibition of monocyte chemotactic protein-1 synthesis by statins. Lab Invest, 80, 1095–1100.

Rosenson, R.S., and Tangney, C.C. (1998). Antiatherothrombotic properties of statins: Implications for cardiovascular event reduction. JAMA, 279, 1643–1650.

Rosenson, R.S., Tangney, C.C., and Casey, L.C. (1999). Inhibition of proinflammatory cytokine production by pravastatin. Lancet, 353, 983–984.

Ross, R. (1999). Ahterosclerosis – an inflammatory disease. N Engl J Med, 340, 115–126.

Rudich, S.M., Mongini, P.K., Perez, R.V., and Katznelson, S. (1998). HMG-CoA reductase inhibitors pravastatin and simvastatin inhibit human b-lymphocyte activation. Transplant Proc, 30, 992–995.

Scalia, R., Gooszen, M.E., Jones, S.P., Hoffmeyer, M., Rimmer, D.M., III, Trocha, S.D., Huang, P.L., Smith, M.B., Lefer, A.M., and Lefer, D.J. (2001). Simvastatin exerts both anti-inflammatory and cardioprotective effects in apolipoprotein E-deficient mice. Circulation, 103, 2598–2603.

Schlienger, R.G., Fedson, D.S., Jick, S.S., Jick, H., and Meier, C.R. (2007). Statins and the risk of pneumonia: A population-based, nested case-control study. Pharmacotherapy, 27, 325–332.

Shi, J., Wang, J., Zheng, H., Ling, W., Joseph, J., Li, D., Mehta, J.L., Ponnappan, U., Lin, P., Fink, L.M., and Hauer-Jensen, M. (2003). Statins increase thrombomodulin expression and function in human endothelial cells by a nitric oxide-dependent mechanism and counteract tumor necrosis factor alpha-induced thrombomodulin downregulation. Blood Coagul Fibrinolysis, 14, 575–585.

Shishehbor, M.H., Brennan, M.L., Aviles, R.J., Fu, X., Penn, M.S., Sprecher, D.L., and Hazen, S.L. (2003). Statins promote potent systemic antioxidant effects through specific inflammatory pathways. Circulation, 108, 426–431.

Steiner, S., Speidl, W.S., Pleiner, J., Seidinger, D., Zorn, G., Kaun, C., Wojta, J., Huber, K., Minar, E., Wolzt, M., and Kopp, C.W. (2005). Simvastatin blunts endotoxin-induced tissue factor in vivo. Circulation, 111, 1841–1846.

Strandberg, T.E., Vanhanen, H., and Tikkanen, M.J. (1999). Effect of statins on C-reactive protein in patients with coronary artery disease. Lancet, 353, 118–119.

Terblanche, M., Almog, Y., Rosenson, R.S., Smith, T.S., and Hackam, D.G. (2007). Statins and sepsis: Multiple modifications at multiple levels. Lancet Infect Dis, 7, 358–368.

Thomsen, R.W., Hundborg, H.H., Johnsen, S.P., Pedersen, L., Sorensen, H.T., Schonheyder, H.C., and Lervang, H.H. (2006). Statin use and mortality within 180 days after bacteremia: A population-based cohort study. Crit Care Med, 34, 1080–1086.

Vincent, J.L., de Mendonca, A., Cantraine, F., Moreno, R., Takala, J., Suter, P.M., Sprung, C.L., Colardyn, F., and Blecher, S. (1998). Use of the sofa score to assess the incidence of organ dysfunction/failure in intensive care units: Results of a multicenter, prospective study. Working group on "Sepsis-related problems" of the European Society of Intensive Care Medicine. Crit Care Med, 26, 1793–1800.

Wang, H.R., Li, J.J., Huang, C.X., and Jiang, H. (2005). Fluvastatin inhibits the expression of tumor necrosis factor-alpha and activation of nuclear factor-kappa b in human endothelial cells stimulated by C-reactive protein. Clin Chim Acta, 353, 53–60.

Weis, M., Pehlivanli, S., Meiser, B.M., and von Scheidt, W. (2001). Simvastatin treatment is associated with improvement in coronary endothelial function and decreased cytokine activation in patients after heart transplantation. J Am Coll Cardiol, 38, 814–818.

Yamamoto, A., Hoshi, K., and Ichihara, K. (1998). Fluvastatin, an inhibitor of 3-hydroxy-3-methylglutaryl-CoA reductase, scavenges free radicals and inhibits lipid peroxidation in rat liver microsomes. Eur J Pharmacol, 361, 143–149.

Yang, K.C., Chien, J.Y., Tseng, W.K., Hsueh, P.R., Yu, C.J., and Wu, C.C. (2007). Statins do not improve short-term survival in an oriental population with sepsis. Am J Emerg Med, 25, 494–501.

Yoshida, M., Sawada, T., Ishii, H., Gerszten, R.E., Rosenzweig, A., Gimbrone, M.A., Jr., Yasukochi, Y., and Numano, F. (2001). HMG-CoA reductase inhibitor modulates monocyte-endothelial cell interaction under physiological flow conditions in vitro: Involvement of rho GTPase-dependent mechanism. Arterioscler Thromb Vasc Biol, 21, 1165–1171.

Chapter 3
The Genetics of Sepsis: The Promise, the Progress and the Pitfalls

Grant W. Waterer

3.1 Introduction

Physicians are used to taking a family history of cardiovascular disease because of the known significant hereditary risk; yet the familial risk of dying from infection is even greater than that for atherosclerotic disease (Sorensen et al. 1988). There is certainly no doubt that genetic differences impact on the risk of developing or dying from infection. Obvious but rare examples include selective immunoglobulin deficiencies, complement deficiencies, and neutrophil function abnormalities. Genetic factors may also be protective, such as with sickle cell trait and malaria or mutations conferring resistance to human immunodeficiency virus infection.

Much more subtle differences in immune responses are now being described, usually as the result of one or more single nucleotide polymorphisms (SNP) in a gene. Rather than causing the failure of production of a protein or the production of a nonfunctional protein, SNPs are usually associated with changes in the rate of transcription, producing a much less severe phenotype than the classical examples of genetic defects mentioned above. It is now being appreciated that for many complex diseases, such as sepsis, the ultimate phenotype is the result of the interaction of genetic differences across many loci, not the dominant effect of a few key mutations.

As seen in Fig. 3.1, since the mid 1990s, an increasing body of literature has focused on the role that gene polymorphisms in key inflammatory genes play in sepsis. Indeed, with advances in knowledge of the human genome, greater understanding of the inflammatory response, and the development of high throughput genotyping technologies, so many genetic associations have been described that discussion of each one is well beyond the scope of this chapter. I will however summarize those findings that have been reported by multiple groups, as well as give an overview of the major groups of genes that have been implicated in genetic predisposition to sepsis and its adverse outcomes.

Despite all this apparent growth in knowledge over the past decade however, to date not one new intervention has been developed as a result of all the genetic studies. As I will discuss, significant limitations in research methodology in published studies combined with the fact that sepsis is not a single disease make it unlikely that we

J. Rello, M.I. Restrepo (eds.) *Sepsis: New Strategies for Management.*
doi:10.1007/978-3-540-79001-3 © Springer-Verlag 2008

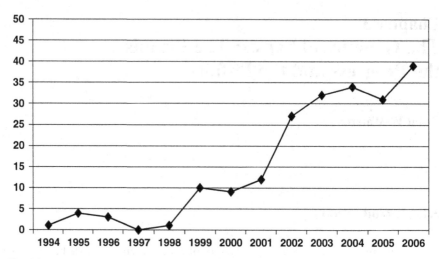

Fig. 3.1 Publications on the genetics of sepsis by year

will see any hope for new interventions in the near future. If we are to truly advance our understanding of sepsis and develop new therapeutic strategies, a substantial change in our current thinking will be required.

3.2 Basic Genetic Terminology

Some basic knowledge of genetic terminology is essential to decipher the sepsis-genetics literature and indeed many apparent contradictions have arisen due to terminology errors. A variety of mutations can occur in DNA, some of which leading to the change in function or production of a gene product. The simplest change is the substitution of one nucleotide for another, a SNP. A number of other mutations occur including the deletion or insertion of one or more nucleotides, including the insertion of multiple repeating sequences, sometimes called a microsatellite.

A region of DNA coding for a protein product is called an exon. Introns are the noncoding regions of DNA separating exons. Most genes consist of several exons and introns. The rate at which genes are transcribed is controlled by a variety of nuclear proteins that bind to different areas of DNA in the 5′ (upstream) region from the first exon. The segment of DNA controlling the regulation of transcription of a gene is also known as the promoter region.

When mutations occur in an exon they may lead to a change in the protein structure of the gene product (nonsynonymous mutation) or they may leave the protein product unchanged (synonymous mutation). When the change occurs in a promoter region, this may alter the binding of a transcription-activating or -suppressing factor, altering the rate of transcription of the gene. Although introns have been considered to be "junk DNA" and therefore mutations are likely to be of little biological importance, it is now appreciated that polymorphisms within introns can affect gene regulation, particularly when they are at the intron–exon boundary (Rohrer and Conely 1998; Meloni et al. 1998; Webb et al. 2003; Lenasi et al. 2006).

Most of the confusion in genetic studies is around the labeling of SNPs. Initially SNPs were assayed by amplifying up the region of DNA with the mutation by polymerase chain reaction and then using an enzyme that cut the DNA based on whether the polymorphism was present or not. Early in the genetic literature it is therefore common to see SNPs referred to by the gene and the enzyme used, for example, the tumor necrosis factor (TNF) NcoI polymorphism (subsequently known as TNF-308).

As it rapidly became apparent that there were often multiple sites within a gene that could be cleaved by the same enzyme, this nomenclature was abandoned in favor of using the nucleotide position relative to the start of the transcription site for the gene (e.g., TNF-308, TNF-238, TNF+1850, etc). This nomenclature dominated the literature for nearly a decade as it is intuitively easy to understand and the number system gives an idea of what the functional significance of the polymorphism is likely to be (e.g., a negative value places it most likely in the promoter region, a positive value in an intron or an exon). When a mutation resulted in an amino acid change in the protein, an alternative nomenclature was often substituted to reflect this (e.g., Toll-like receptor 4 (TLR4) Thr399Ile indicates that an isoleucine is substituted for a threonine at amino acid position 399).

Unfortunately, differences in calculation of the transcription start site for genes led to increasing confusion – for example, the lymphotoxin alpha (LTA, formally known as tumor necrosis factor beta) polymorphism, reported by Stuber and colleagues (1996) as a risk factor for sepsis, was variably reported as LTA+249, LTA+250, LTA+251, and LTA+252. With hundreds of thousands if not millions of polymorphisms now described, the accepted practice for indicating the exact polymorphism being described is currently the reference sequence number (rs#) on the National Institutes of Health database (e.g., the TNF NcoI or -308 polymorphism is officially rs1800629). While all publications should reference the rs#, it is likely that older terminology will continue to be used for sometime until it is more familiar.

A final problem with nomenclature that needs to be discussed is the labeling of individual alleles. There was a convention commonly seen in early genetics literature that the most common allele in the population studies was referred to as allele 1 (or A), the second most common allele 2 (or B), and so on (i.e., TNF-308 allele 1). As allele frequencies can vary significantly between populations, this has the potential to lead to considerable confusion and they should instead be referred to by the nucleotide carriage (e.g., TNF-308 A or TNF-308 G) or the number of nucleotide repeats.

3.3 Studies of Genetic Influence on the Inflammatory Response

Genetic polymorphisms with potential influences on the inflammatory response have been identified in a variety of antigen recognition, pro- and anti-inflammatory cytokines. All of these polymorphisms are candidates for studies in genetic influences on sepsis and its outcomes, and Table 3.1 summarizes studies that have been published.

Table 3.1 An enormous number of genes have been identified as having potentially important polymorphic sites

Antigen recognition	Pro-inflammatory	Anti-inflammatory	Coagulation and tissue repair pathways
CD14 (Baier et al 2006; Barber et al 2006; Gibot et al 2002; Heesen et al 2002; Nakada et al 2005; Skinner et al 2005; Temple et al 2003)	TNF (Barber et al 2006; Calvano et al 2003; Gong et al 2005; Gordon et al 2004; Hedberg et al 2004; Majetschak et al 1999; Mira et al 1999; Nakada et al 2005; Nuntayanuwat et al 1999; O'Keefe et al 2002; Stuber et al 1995; Waterer et al 2001; Westendorp et al 1997)	IL-10 (Baier et al 2006; Balding et al 2003; Gallagher et al 2003; Gong et al 2006; Lowe et al 2003; Nakada et al 2005; Schaaf et al 2003; Shu et al 2003; Stanilova et al 2006; Sutherland et al 2005; Wattanathum et al 2005; Westendorp et al 1997)	Fibrinogen-beta (Manocha et al 2007)
TLR4 (Barber et al 2006; Lorenz et al 2002; Nakada et al 2005; Skinner et al 2005), TLR2 (Skinner et al 2005), TLR5 (Hawn et al 2003)	IL-1β (Watanabe et al 2005), IL-6 (Baier et al 2006; Balding et al 2003; Barber et al 2006; Schluter et al 2002; Sutherland et al 2005), IL-18 (Stassen et al 2003)	IL-1 receptor antagonist (Arnalich et al 2002; Balding et al 2003; Fang et al 1999)	Protein-C (Walley & Russell 2007)
Lippopolysaccharide binding protein (Barber & O'Keefe 2003; Hubacek et al 2001)	CXCL2 (Flores et al 2006)	Heat shock protein 70 complex (Schroder et al 2003; Waterer et al 2003)	Vascular endothelial growth factor (Zhai et al 2007)
IgG2 receptor (also the C-reactive protein receptor) (Yuan et al 2003)	Lymphotoxin alpha (Calvano et al 2003; Majetschak et al 1999; Rauchschwalbe et al 2004; Stuber et al 1996; Waterer et al 2001)		Factor V (Weiler etal 2004; Yan & Nelson 2004)
Myeloid differentiation protein-2 (MD-2) (Gu et al 2007)	Macrophage migration inhibition factor (MIF) (Gao et al 2007)		Apolipoprotein-E (Moretti et al 2005)
C-reactive protein (Eklund et al 2006)	Pre-B cell colony stimulating factor (PBEF) (Bajwa et al 2007; Ye et al 2005)		Plasminogen activator inhibitor-1 (Binder et al 2007a; Binder et al 2007b; Geishofer et al 2005a; Geishofer et al 2005b; Hermans et al 1999)
Mannose-binding lectin (Garred et al 2003; Gong et al 2007; Gordon et al 2006; Kronborg et al 2002; Roy et al 2002)	IRAK-1 (Arcaroli et al 2006)		
Surfactant-proteins (Gong et al 2004; Quasney et al 2004)			

As there is substantial overlap between the functions of many cytokines, and frequently multiple antagonists for any given agonist, there is a significant ability to compensate for a certain amount of divergence in production of individual cytokines. Therefore, for a single mutation to influence the outcome of an inflammatory response, it must markedly alter the production or function of a critical inflammatory protein. While possible, the more likely scenario already discussed is the inheritance of multiple mutations in multiple proteins, each leading to small changes in production or function, interacting to lead to a net serious deleterious effect.

While a complete review of all polymorphisms described within the immune response genes is well beyond the scope of this chapter, the following section will discuss some of the key findings in various components of the immune response.

3.3.1 Pattern Recognition Molecules

Once the microorganism reaches the lower respiratory tract, organization of the innate immune system allows recognition of molecular patterns that are not found in humans. These so-called pattern recognition molecules (PRMs) can then initiate opsonization and lysis of microorganisms, enhance clearance by alveolar macrophages and neutrophils, as well as initiate an antibody response.

3.3.1.1 Collectins

Collectins are a family of PRMs that include surfactant proteins A and D and mannose-binding lectin (MBL), with a large degree of sequence homology present between the three compounds. MBL is the plasma form and has independent ability to activate the complement system. Conservation of MBL in various species suggests that it plays an important role in innate immunity. Several mutations in the gene itself or in the promoter region can lead to little or no serum MBL. MBL polymorphisms were found to be a risk factor for severe sepsis in adults (Garred et al. 2003), and the incidence of homozygous variant alleles in the introns was twice as common in patients with invasive pneumococcal disease in one study (Roy et al. 2002) but not in other studies (Kronborg et al. 2002). Some of the conflicting reports may be due to looking at only a limited number of polymorphisms instead of all variants or because of the significant variability in frequency of the variant alleles in different racial/ethnic groups.

3.3.1.2 Toll-Like Receptors (TLRs)

Another class of PRMs is the toll-like receptors (TLRs), human transmembrane signaling proteins equivalent to the Drosophila toll molecule found to be important in immunity against bacteria and fungi. Ten TLRs have been identified in humans, each with different affinities for antigens of different microorganisms (Beutler 2002). Most of the initial clinical research has focused on genetic variants of TLR4 essential for recognition of LPS. Variants in the TLR4 gene appear to increase the risk of serious gram-negative infections and sepsis (Lorenz et al. 2002). TLR4 is however unlikely to play an important role in gram-positive sepsis as TLR2 is more specific for recognition of peptidoglycans from gram-positive bacteria. Rare TLR2 polymorphisms have been described as increasing the risk of gram-positive infections (Sutherland et al. 2005b) and a TLR5 mutation has been associated with an increased risk of legionella infection (Hawn et al. 2003).

3.3.1.3   Other Endotoxin Recognition Molecules

Other key components of endotoxin recognition and signaling that have been studied as potential genetic risk factors for sepsis other than TLR4 include CD14, Myeloid differentiation protein-2 (MD-2), and lippopollysaccharide binding protein (LBP). The results for LBP gene mutations have been far from conclusive with conflicting reports (Hubacek et al. 2001; Barber and O'Keefe 2003). In contrast, studies of CD14 polymorphism have produced more consistent findings. A relatively common CD14 mutation is associated with higher soluble CD14 levels and an increased risk of septic shock (71% vs. 48%, $p = 0.008$) (Gibot et al. 2002). The same polymorphism is also associated with greater TNF production after endotoxin stimulation of peripheral blood mononuclear cells in healthy adults (Temple et al. 2003a). Mutations in MD2 have also been linked with an increased risk of sepsis (Gu et al. 2007).

3.3.1.4   Immunoglobulin Receptors

Genetic variation in adaptive immunity may also play a role in sepsis. A variant in the CD32 (FcγRII) subclass is associated with decreased binding of the IgG2 subclass (Yuan et al. 2003). Patients homozygous for the FcγRIIa-R131 allele were more common in patients with bacteremic pneumococcal pneumonia, nonbacteremic pneumonia, or healthy controls (Yee et al. 1997). This association has been confirmed in a separate case–control study (Yuan et al. 2003). Patients with the FcγRIIa-R131 allele also appear to be more susceptible to meningococcal meningitis, as well as more susceptible to severe complications such as septic shock (van der Pol et al. 2001).

3.3.2   Inflammatory/Anti-inflammatory Response

3.3.2.1   Tumor Necrosis Factor (TNF)

Tumor necrosis factor (TNF) is critical to the immune response to infection (Beutler and Grau 1993), and a key driver to the development of septic shock (Bochud and

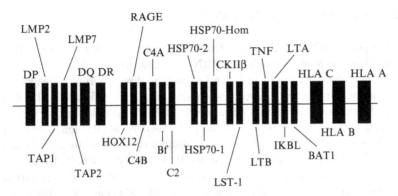

Fig. 3.2 The immunologically rich MHC region containing TNF

Calandra 2003). The TNF gene is also highly polymorphic, leading to a large array of association studies in literally hundreds of different diseases. Complicating matters further, TNF is in the immunology-gene rich area of chromosome 6 (Fig. 3.2).

The TNF-308 polymorphism is by far the most comprehensively studied genetic variation in immune response that has been reported. Carriers of the A allele (G is the more common nucleotide in all populations studied) has been associated with an increased risk of death from a variety of infectious diseases, including septic shock (Azim et al. 2007; Calvano et al. 2003; Cirpriano et al. 2005; Nakada et al. 2005; Schueller et al. 2006; Mira et al. 1999; O'Keefe et al. 2002). However, other investigators have not found a significant association between the TNF-308 A allele and death from or risk of sepsis (Stuber et al. 1995; Waterer et al. 2001). The TNF-308 polymorphism is in significant linkage disequilibrium with multiple other polymorphic sites within TNF itself and in the wider MHC region. This extensive linkage disequilibrium may not only explain the disparate findings between studies, but also why after over a decade of research, there is no agreement on whether or not the different TNF-308 alleles result in differential production of TNF (Bayley et al. 2004).

3.3.2.2 Lymphotoxin Alpha (LTA)

Adenine homozygosity of LTA+252, a G to A transition in the first intron of LTA, has been associated with increased TNF production and was one of the first genetic factors identified as a potential risk factor for death from septic shock (Stuber et al. 1996; Majetschak et al. 1999). The same genotype has also been associated with an increased risk of septic shock in patients with pneumonia (Waterer et al. 2001). In the latter study, it was interesting that respiratory failure correlated with the GG genotype (Waterer et al. 2001), the opposite of the association for shock. However, given LTA+252 is located in an intron, the association with variable TNF production is most likely due to linkage disequilibrium with other variant alleles in the TNF, LTA, or other nearby genes.

3.3.2.3 Interleukin – 1 (IL-1) Family

The IL-1 gene family includes the potent inflammatory agonists IL-1α and IL-1β, and the IL-1 receptor antagonist (IL-1RN), adjacent to each other on the same chromosome and therefore there is marked linkage disequilibrium between poly-morphisms within the three genes. Two SNPs, the IL-1β+3953 and −511, which have both been suggested to influence levels of IL-1β (Pociot et al. 1992), were associated with increased risk of death from meningococcal infection in one cohort study (Read et al. 2000) but not with susceptibility to or outcome from septic shock (Fang et al. 1999). In contrast, variants of the IL-1RN gene have been demonstrated to have an excess mortality in septic patients in three sepsis studies in different ethnic groups (Fang et al. 1999; Arnalich et al. 2002; Ma et al. 2002; Turner et al. 1997), although these studies did not assess potential coinherited polymorphisms in IL-1α and IL-1β making it difficult to be sure the associations observed were attributable to the IL-1-RN variants.

3.3.2.4 Interleukin 10 (IL-10)

IL-10 is another highly polymorphic gene. Three promoter polymorphisms (-1082/-819/-592) have been extensively studied and different -819/-592 haplotypes associated with variable IL-10 production (Turner et al. 1997). The effect of the IL-10 haplotype however appears to be pathogen-dependent, with a significantly different genotype–phenotype relationship observed depending on whether the stimulus is gram-positive or gram-negative (Temple et al. 2003b).

Several case–control studies have suggested that carriage of the IL-10 -1082 G allele is a significant risk factor for adverse outcome in patients with pneumonia (Gallagher et al. 2003; Schaaf et al. 2003). Case–control studies also suggest that the IL-10-1082 G allele is a risk factor for death from septic shock (Stanilolva et al. 2006), and a risk factor for multiorgan dysfunction after major trauma (Schroder et al. 2004).

3.3.2.5 Heat Shock Protein

While intracellular heat shock proteins (HSPs) principally play a cytoprotective role, extracellular HSP70 can induce a proinflammatory response through TLR2 and TLR4 via a CD14-dependent mechanism. As shown in Fig. 3.2, the HSP-70 locus is also close to the TNF and LTA loci. A significant association between the A allele of HSPA1B+1267 and septic shock has been demonstrated in an extension of the pneumonia study mentioned above (Waterer et al. 2003), which was even stronger than that of the LTA+252. This stronger association, combined with functional studies showing that the HSP-A1B polymorphism was associated with variable HSP-70 production and TNF production (Temple et al. 2004) strongly suggests that this is the "real" cause of the associations described with LTA+252.

3.3.3 Coagulation Pathway Proteins

An extremely large number of polymorphisms have now been described within the pro- and anticoagulant hemostatic pathways, many of which being suggested to influence coagulation. With the increase in interest in the role of coagulation in the outcome of severe sepsis due to the success of activated protein-C (Bernard et al. 2001), it is not surprising that there has been an increase in interest in genetic differences in coagulation pathways and the risk of sepsis.

An insertion/deletion polymorphism in plasminogen activation inhibitor (PAI)-1 is associated with variation in serum PAI-1 levels (Ye et al. 1995) and has been suggested as a significant risk factor for mortality in children with meningococcal disease (Binder et al. 2007; Geishofer et al. 2005; Haralambous et al. 2003). One study in adults also suggests that the same polymorphism is a risk factor for death from septic shock in caucasians (Garcia-Segarra et al. 2007; Hermans et al. 1999).

3.4 Problems with Genetic Studies in Sepsis

What explains the diversity of findings in studies of genetic influence on sepsis? There is no doubt that simple genotyping error, particularly before the advent of highly automated platforms, is a significant source of error in polymorphism studies (Clark and Baudouin 2006; Sutherland and Russell 2005; Peters et al. 2003). As early studies typically contained less than 100 subjects, even a few genotyping errors, particularly with rare genotypes, can have a dramatic impact on statistical significance. It is important that all genetic studies perform and report adequate quality control measures to ensure genotyping is accurate.

The problems of linkage disequilibrium have been mentioned several times. As the human genome is so highly polymorphic, the likelihood that any studied polymorphism is the "real" site of significance is low. Newer genetic methods, particularly genotyping multiple nearby SNPs to determine the "length" of DNA associated with the clinical outcome (known as haplotype mapping) are a significant aid in trying to determine the key genetic area.

As already discussed with TNF-308, actually proving that a polymorphism is functionally significant is a very difficult task unless the polymorphism results in a change in the protein structure. There are numerous examples of different groups claiming that a polymorphism is (or is not) functionally important based on different stimuli, cell types, and sample timing.

Compounding the difficulty in finding associations is that even if a polymorphism results in a functional change in the production of a key protein, this could have both detrimental and beneficial effects depending on the outcome concerned. For example, a propensity to greater TNF may be protective in reducing the risk of developing infection; however, if pneumonia becomes established, it may predispose to a greater risk of acute respiratory distress syndrome or septic shock.

Another problem limiting the development of new therapeutic strategies arising from genetic studies is the timing of the influence of the polymorphism. For example, TNF polymorphisms may be important in the risk of septic shock; however, as the failed randomized controlled trials of anti-TNF antibodies demonstrated, once septic shock is established, modifying TNF production has no benefit. Many genetic factors predisposing to an initial event are likely to suffer from the same problem given that patients typically present well after infection has been established.

Finally, the number of polymorphisms already reported as being "important" is significant. Studies that address only one or two polymorphisms without studying previously reported polymorphisms so that the new findings can be put into a relative context do little to advance our knowledge (Waterer 2007). Unfortunately, given the issues with multiple testing, the sample size to sort out the relative contributions of all these polymorphisms is in tens of thousands.

3.5 Summary

There is an increasing array of polymorphisms in diverse inflammatory genes that have been identified as candidates to explain genetic variability in susceptibility to septic shock and its adverse outcomes. Unfortunately, to date, the ever-expanding volume of publications has not led to any new therapeutic insights. The failure to advance to the "next step" is due in part to failings of published studies, but mostly because of the fact that sepsis is almost certainly the result of hundreds, if not thousands, of mutations that each contribute in a small way to a very complex phenotype. Future studies will hopefully learn from the mistakes of the past and realize the enormous promise of genetic studies.

References

Arcaroli, J., E. Silva, J. Maloney, Q. He, D. Svetkauskaite, J. Murphy, and E. Abraham. 2006. Variant IRAK-1 haplotype is associated with increased nuclear factor-kappaB activation and worse outcomes in sepsis. *Am J Respir Crit Care Med* 173:1335–41.

Arnalich, F., D. Lopez-Maderuelo, R. Codoceo, J. Lopez, L. M. Solis-Garrido, C. Capiscol, C. Fernandez-Capitan, R. Madero, and C. Montiel. 2002. Interleukin-1 receptor antagonist gene polymorphism and mortality in patients with severe sepsis. *Clin Exp Immunol* 127:331–6.

Azim, K., R. McManus, K. Brophy, A. Ryan, D. Kelleher, and J. V. Reynolds. 2007. Genetic polymorphisms and the risk of infection following esophagectomy. Positive association with TNF-alpha gene -308 genotype. *Ann Surg* 246:122–8.

Baier, R., J. Loggins, and K. Yanamandra. 2006. IL-10, IL-6 and CD14 polymorphisms and sepsis outcome in ventilated very low birth weight infants. *BMC Med* 12:10–12.

Bajwa, E., C. Yu, M. Gong, B. Thompson, and D. Christiani. 2007. Pre-B-cell colony-enhancing factor gene polymorphisms and risk of acute respiratory distress syndrome. *Crit Care Med* 35:1290–5.

Balding, J., C. M. Healy, W. J. Livingstone, B. White, L. Mynett-Johnson, M. Cafferkey, and O. P. Smith. 2003. Genomic polymorphic profiles in an Irish population with meningococcaemia: is it possible to predict severity and outcome of disease? *Genes Immun* 4:533–40.

Barber, R., L. Chang, B. D. Arnoldo, G. Purdue, J. Hunt, J. Horton, and C. Aragaki. 2006. Innate immunity SNPs are associated with risk for severe sepsis after burn injury. *Clin Med Res* 4:250–5.

Barber, R. C., and G. E. O'Keefe. 2003. Characterization of a single nucleotide polymorphism in the lipopolysaccharide binding protein and its association with sepsis. *Am J Respir Crit Care Med* 167:1316–20.

Bayley, J. P., T. H. Ottenhoff, and C. L. Verweij. 2004. Is there a future for TNF promoter polymorphisms? *Genes Immun* 5:315–29.

Bernard, G. R., J. L. Vincent, P. F. Laterre, S. P. LaRosa, J. F. Dhainaut, A. Lopez-Rodriguez, J. S. Steingrub, G. E. Garber, J. D. Helterbrand, E. W. Ely, and C. J. Fisher, Jr. 2001. Efficacy and safety of recombinant human activated protein C for severe sepsis. *N Engl J Med* 344:699–709.

Beutler, B. 2002. Toll-like receptors: how they work and what they do. *Curr Opin Hematol* 9:2–10.

Beutler, B., and G. E. Grau. 1993. Tumor necrosis factor in the pathogenesis of infectious diseases. *Crit Care Med* 21(10 Suppl):S423–35.

Binder, A., G. Endler, M. Muller, C. Mannhalter, and W. Zenz. 2007. 4G4G genotype of the plasminogen activator inhibitor-1 promoter polymorphism associates with disseminated intravascular coagulation in children with systemic meningococcemia. *J Thromb Haemost* 5:2049–54.

Bochud, P. Y., and T. Calandra. 2003. Pathogenesis of sepsis: new concepts and implications for future treatment. *BMJ* 326(7383):262–6.

Calvano, J. E., J. Y. Um, D. M. Agnese, S. J. Hahm, A. Kumar, S. M. Coyle, S. E. Calvano, and S. F. Lowry. 2003. Influence of the TNF-alpha and TNF-beta polymorphisms upon infectious risk and outcome in surgical intensive care patients. *Surg Infect (Larchmt)* 4:163–9.

Cipriano, C., C. Caruso, D. Lio, R. Giacconi, M. Malavolta, E. Muti, N. Gasparini, C. Franceschi, and E. Mocchegiani. 2005. The -308G/A polymorphism of TNF-alpha influences immunological parameters in old subjects affected by infectious diseases. *Int J Immunogenet* 32:13–18.

Clark, M., and S. Baudouin. 2006. A systematic review of the quality of genetic association studies in human sepsis. *Intensive Care Med* 32:1679–80.

Eklund, C., R. Huttunen, J. Syrjänen, J. Laine, R. Vuento, and M. Hurme. 2006. Polymorphism of the C-reactive protein gene is associated with mortality in bacteraemia. *Scand J Infect Dis* 38(11–12):1069–73.

Fang, X. M., S. Schroder, A. Hoeft, and F. Stuber. 1999. Comparison of two polymorphisms of the interleukin-1 gene family: interleukin-1 receptor antagonist polymorphism contributes to susceptibility to severe sepsis. *Crit Care Med* 27:1330–4.

Flores, C., N. Maca-Meyer, L. Pérez-Méndez, R. Sangüesa, E. Espinosa, A. Muriel, J. Blanco, J. Villar, G. group, and G.- S. group. 2006. A CXCL2 tandem repeat promoter polymorphism is associated with susceptibility to severe sepsis in the Spanish population. *Genes Immun* 7:141–9.

Gallagher, P. M., G. Lowe, T. Fitzgerald, A. Bella, C. M. Greene, N. G. McElvaney, and S. J. O'Neill. 2003. Association of IL-10 polymorphism with severity of illness in community acquired pneumonia. *Thorax* 58:154–6.

Gao, L., C. Flores, S. Fan-Ma, E. Miller, J. Moitra, L. Moreno, R. Wadgaonkar, B. Simon, R. Brower, J. Sevransky, R. Tuder, J. Maloney, M. Moss, C. Shanholtz, C. Yates, G. Meduri, S. Ye, K. Barnes, and J. Garcia. 2007. Macrophage migration inhibitory factor in acute lung injury: expression, biomarker, and associations. *Transl Res* 150:18–29.

Garcia-Segarra, G., G. Espinosa, D. Tassies, J. Oriola, J. Aibar, A. Bove, P. Castro, J. C. Reverter, and J. M. Nicolas. 2007. Increased mortality in septic shock with the 4G/4G genotype of plasminogen activator inhibitor 1 in patients of white descent. *Intensive Care Med* 33:1354–62.

Garred, P., J. Strøm, L. Quist, E. Taaning, and H. Madsen. 2003. Association of mannose-binding lectin polymorphisms with sepsis and fatal outcome, in patients with systemic inflammatory response syndrome. *J Infect Dis* 188:1394–1403.

Geishofer, G., A. Binder, M. Muller, B. Zohrer, B. Resch, W. Muller, J. Faber, A. Finn, G. Endler, C. Mannhalter, W. Zenz, and C. E. M. G. S. Group. 2005. 4G/5G promoter polymorphism in the plasminogen-activator-inhibitor-1 gene in children with systemic meningococcaemia. *Eur J Pediatr* 164:486–90.

Gibot, S., A. Cariou, L. Drouet, M. Rossignol, and L. Ripoll. 2002. Association between a genomic polymorphism within the CD14 locus and septic shock susceptibility and mortality rate. *Crit Care Med* 30:969–73.

Gong, M. N., Z. Wei, L. L. Xu, D. P. Miller, B. T. Thompson, and D. C. Christiani. 2004. Polymorphism in the surfactant protein-B gene, gender, and the risk of direct pulmonary injury and ARDS. *Chest* 125:203–11.

Gong, M. N., W. Zhou, P. L. Williams, B. T. Thompson, L. Pothier, P. Boyce, and D. C. Christiani. 2005. -308GA and TNFB polymorphisms in acute respiratory distress syndrome. *Eur Respir J* 26:382–9.

Gong, M. N., B. T. Thompson, P. L. Williams, W. Zhou, M. Z. Wang, L. Pothier, and D. C. Christiani. 2006. Interleukin-10 polymorphism in position -1082 and acute respiratory distress syndrome. *Eur Respir J* 27:674–81.

Gong, M. N., W. Zhou, P. L. Williams, B. T. Thompson, L. Pothier, and D. C. Christiani. 2007. Polymorphisms in the mannose binding lectin-2 gene and acute respiratory distress syndrome. *Crit Care Med* 35:48–56.

Gordon, A. C., A. L. Lagan, E. Aganna, L. Cheung, C. J. Peters, M. F. McDermott, J. L. Millo, K. I. Welsh, P. Holloway, G. A. Hitman, R. D. Piper, C. S. Garrard, and C. J. Hinds. 2004. TNF and TNFR polymorphisms in severe sepsis and septic shock: a prospective multicentre study. *Genes Immun* 5:631–40.

Gordon, A., U. Waheed, T. Hansen, G. Hitman, C. Garrard, M. Turner, N. Klein, S. Brett, and C. Hinds. 2006. Mannose-binding lectin polymorphisms in severe sepsis: relationship to levels, incidence, and outcome. *Shock* 25:88–93.

Gu, W., Y. Shan, J. Zhou, D. Jiang, L. Zhang, D. Du, Z. Wang, and J. Jiang. 2007. Functional significance of gene polymorphisms in the promoter of myeloid differentiation-2. *Ann Surg* 246:151–8.

Haralambous, E., M. L. Hibberd, P. W. Hermans, N. Ninis, S. Nadel, and M. Levin. 2003. Role of functional plasminogen-activator-inhibitor-1 4G/5G promoter polymorphism in susceptibility, severity, and outcome of meningococcal disease in Caucasian children. *Crit Care Med* 31:2788–93.

Hawn, T. R., A. Verbon, K. D. Lettinga, L. P. Zhao, S. S. Li, R. J. Laws, S. J. Skerrett, B. Beutler, L. Schroeder, A. Nachman, A. Ozinsky, K. D. Smith, and A. Aderem. 2003. A common dominant TLR5 stop codon polymorphism abolishes flagellin signaling and is associated with susceptibility to legionnaires' disease. *J Exp Med* 198:1563–72.

Hedberg, C. L., K. Adcock, J. Martin, J. Loggins, T. E. Kruger, and R. J. Baier. 2004. Tumor necrosis factor alpha – 308 polymorphism associated with increased sepsis mortality in ventilated very low birth weight infants. *Pediatr Infect Dis J* 23:424–8.

Heesen, M., B. Bloemeke, U. Schade, U. Obertacke, and M. Majetschak. 2002. The -260 C→T promoter polymorphism of the lipopolysaccharide receptor CD14 and severe sepsis in trauma patients. *Intensive Care Med* 28:1161–3.

Hermans, P. W., M. L. Hibberd, R. Booy, O. Daramola, J. A. Hazelzet, R. de Groot, and M. Levin. 1999. 4G/5G promoter polymorphism in the plasminogen-activator-inhibitor-1 gene and outcome of meningococcal disease. Meningococcal Research Group. *Lancet* 354(9178):556–60.

Hubacek, J. A., F. Stuber, D. Frohlich, M. Book, S. Wetegrove, M. Ritter, G. Rothe, and G. Schmitz. 2001. Gene variants of the bactericidal/permeability increasing protein and lipopolysaccharide binding protein in sepsis patients: gender-specific genetic predisposition to sepsis. *Crit Care Med* 29:557–61.

Kronborg, G., N. Weis, H. Madsen, S. Pedersen, C. Wejse, H. Nielsen, et al. 2002. Variant mannose-binding lectin alleles are not associated with susceptibility to or outcome of invasive pneumococcal infection in randomly included patients. *J Infect Dis* 185:1517–20.

Lenasi, T., B. M. Peterlin, and P. Dovc. 2006. Distal regulation of alternative splicing by splicing enhancer in equine beta-casein intron 1. *RNA* 12:498–507.

Lorenz, E., J. Mira, K. Frees, and D. Schwartz. 2002. Relevance of mutations in the TLR4 receptor in patients with gram-negative septic shock. *Arch Intern Med* 162:1028–32.

Lowe, P. R., H. F. Galley, A. Abdel-Fattah, and N. R. Webster. 2003. Influence of interleukin-10 polymorphisms on interleukin-10 expression and survival in critically ill patients. *Crit Care Med* 31:34–8.

Ma, P., D. Chen, J. Pan, and B. Du. 2002. Genomic polymorphism within interleukin-1 family cytokines influences the outcome of septic patients. *Zhonghua Yi Xue Za Zhi* 82:1237–41.

Majetschak, M., S. Flohe, U. Obertacke, J. Schroder, K. Staubach, D. Nast-Kolb, F. U. Schade, and F. Stuber. 1999. Relation of a TNF gene polymorphism to severe sepsis in trauma patients. *Ann Surg* 230:207–14.

Manocha, S., J. Russell, A. Sutherland, A. Wattanathum, and K. Walley. 2007. Fibrinogen-beta gene haplotype is associated with mortality in sepsis. *J Infect* 54:572–7.

Meloni, R., V. Albanese, P. Ravassard, F. Treilhou, and J. Mallet. 1998. A tetranucleotide polymorphic microsatellite, located in the first intron of the tyrosine hydroxylase gene, acts as a transcription regulatory element in vitro. *Hum Mol Genet* 7:423–8.

Mira, J. P., A. Cariou, F. Grall, C. Delclaux, M. R. Losser, F. Heshmati, C. Cheval, M. Monchi, J. L. Teboul, F. Riche, G. Leleu, L. Arbibe, A. Mignon, M. Delpech, and J. F. Dhainaut. 1999. Association of TNF2, a TNF-alpha promoter polymorphism, with septic shock susceptibility and mortality: a multicenter study. *JAMA* 282:561–8.

Moretti, E. W., R. W. Morris, M. Podgoreanu, D. A. Schwinn, M. F. Newman, E. Bennett, V. G. Moulin, U. U. Mba, and D. T. Laskowitz. 2005. APOE polymorphism is associated with risk of severe sepsis in surgical patients. *Crit Care Med* 33:2521–6.

Nakada, T. A., H. Hirasawa, S. Oda, H. Shiga, K. I. Matsuda, M. Nakamura, E. Watanabe, R. Abe, M. Hatano, and T. Tokuhisa. 2005. Influence of toll-like receptor 4, CD14, tumor necrosis factor, and interleukine-10 gene polymorphisms on clinical outcome in Japanese critically ill patients. *J Surg Res* 129:322–8.

Nuntayanuwat, S., T. Dharakul, W. Chaowagul, and S. Songsivilai. 1999. Polymorphism in the promoter region of tumor necrosis factor-alpha gene is associated with severe meliodosis. *Hum Immunol* 60:979–83.

O'Keefe, G. E., D. L. Hybki, and R. S. Munford. 2002. The G→A single nucleotide polymorphism at the -308 position in the tumor necrosis factor-alpha promoter increases the risk for severe sepsis after trauma. *J Trauma* 52:817–25; discussion 825–6.

Peters, D. L., R. C. Barber, E. M. Flood, H. R. Garner, and G. E. O'Keefe. 2003. Methodologic quality and genotyping reproducibility in studies of tumor necrosis factor -308 ****G→A single nucleotide polymorphism and bacterial sepsis: implications for studies of complex traits. *Crit Care Med* 31:1691–6.

Pociot, F., J. Molvig, L. Wogensen, H. Worsaae, and J. Nerup. 1992. A TaqI polymorphism in the human interleukin-1 beta (IL-1 beta) gene correlates with IL-1 beta secretion in vitro. *Eur J Clin Invest* 22:396–402.

Quasney, M. W., G. W. Waterer, M. K. Dahmer, G. K. Kron, Q. Zhang, L. A. Kessler, and R. G. Wunderink. 2004. Association between surfactant protein B+1580 polymorphism and the risk of respiratory failure in adults with community-acquired pneumonia. *Crit Care Med* 32:1115–19.

Rauchschwalbe, S. K., T. Maseizik, U. Mittelkotter, B. Schluter, C. Patzig, A. Thiede, and H. B. Reith. 2004. Effect of the LT-alpha (+250 G/A) polymorphism on markers of inflammation and clinical outcome in critically ill patients. *J Trauma* 56:815–22.

Read, R. C., N. J. Camp, F. S. di Giovine, R. Borrow, E. B. Kaczmarski, A. G. Chaudhary, A. J. Fox, and G. W. Duff. 2000. An interleukin-1 genotype is associated with fatal outcome of meningococcal disease. *J Infect Dis* 182:1557–60.

Rohrer, J., and M. E. Conley. 1998. Transcriptional regulatory elements within the first intron of Bruton's tyrosine kinase. *Blood* 91:214–21.

Roy, S., K. Knox, S. Segal, D. Griffiths, C. Moore, K. Welsh, et al. 2002. MBL genotype and risk of invasive pneumococcal disease: a case–control study. *Lancet* 359(9317):1569–73.

Schaaf, B. M., F. Boehmke, H. Esnaashari, U. Seitzer, H. Kothe, M. Maass, P. Zabel, and K. Dalhoff. 2003. Pneumococcal septic shock is associated with the interleukin-10-1082 gene promoter polymorphism. *Am J Respir Crit Care Med* 168:476–80.

Schluter, B., C. Raufhake, M. Erren, H. Schotte, F. Kipp, S. Rust, H. Van Aken, G. Assmann, and E. Berendes. 2002. Effect of the interleukin-6 promoter polymorphism (-174 G/C) on the incidence and outcome of sepsis. *Crit Care Med* 30:32–7.

Schroder, O., K. M. Schulte, P. Ostermann, H. D. Roher, A. Ekkernkamp, and R. A. Laun. 2003. Heat shock protein 70 genotypes HSPA1B and HSPA1L influence cytokine concentrations and interfere with outcome after major injury. *Crit Care Med* 31:73–9.

Schroder, O., R. A. Laun, B. Held, A. Ekkernkamp, and K. M. Schulte. 2004. Association of interleukin-10 promoter polymorphism with the incidence of multiple organ dysfunction following major trauma: results of a prospective pilot study. *Shock* 21:306–10.

Schueller, A. C., A. Heep, E. Kattner, M. Kroll, M. Wisbauer, J. Sander, P. Bartmann, and F. Stuber. 2006. Prevalence of two tumor necrosis factor gene polymorphisms in premature infants with early onset sepsis. *Biol Neonate* 90:229–32.

Shu, Q., X. Fang, Q. Chen, and F. Stuber. 2003. IL-10 polymorphism is associated with increased incidence of severe sepsis. *Chin Med J (Engl)* 116:1756–9.

Skinner, N. A., C. M. MacIsaac, J. A. Hamilton, and K. Visvanathan. 2005. Regulation of toll-like receptor (TLR)2 and TLR4 on CD14dimCD16+ monocytes in response to sepsis-related antigens. *Clin Exp Immunol* 141:270–8.

Sorensen, T. I., G. G. Nielsen, P. K. Andersen, and T. W. Teasdale. 1988. Genetic and environmental influences on premature death in adult adoptees. *N Engl J Med* 318:727–32.

Stanilova, S. A., L. D. Miteva, Z. T. Karakolev, and C. S. Stefanov. 2006. Interleukin-10-1082 promoter polymorphism in association with cytokine production and sepsis susceptibility. *Intensive Care Med* 32:260–6.

Stassen, N. A., C. M. Breit, L. A. Norfleet, and H. C. Polk, Jr. 2003. IL-18 promoter polymorphisms correlate with the development of post-injury sepsis. *Surgery* 134:351–6.

Stuber, F., I. A. Udalova, M. Book, L. N. Drutskaya, D. V. Kuprash, R. L. Turetskaya, F. U. Schade, and S. A. Nedospasov. 1995. -308 tumor necrosis factor (TNF) polymorphism is not associated with survival in severe sepsis and is unrelated to lipopolysaccharide inducibility of the human TNF promoter. *J Inflamm* 46:42–50.

Stuber, F., M. Petersen, F. Bokelmann, and U. Schade. 1996. A genomic polymorphism within the tumor necrosis factor locus influences plasma tumor necrosis factor-alpha concentrations and outcome of patients with severe sepsis. *Crit Care Med* 24:381–4.

Sutherland, A. M., and J. A. Russell. 2005. Issues with polymorphism analysis in sepsis. *Clin Infect Dis* 41(7 Suppl):S396–402.

Sutherland, A. M., K. R. Walley, and J. A. Russell. 2005a. Polymorphisms in CD14, mannose-binding lectin, and toll-like receptor-2 are associated with increased prevalence of infection in critically ill adults. *Crit Care Med* 33:638–44.

Sutherland, A. M., K. R. Walley, S. Manocha, and J. A. Russell. 2005b. The association of interleukin 6 haplotype clades with mortality in critically ill adults. *Arch Intern Med* 165:75–82.

Temple, S. E., K. Y. Cheong, C. M. Almeida, P. Price, and G. W. Waterer. 2003a. Polymorphisms in lymphotoxin alpha and CD14 genes influence TNF alpha production induced by Gram-positive and Gram-negative bacteria. *Genes Immun* 4:283–8.

Temple, S. E., E. Lim, K. Y. Cheong, C. A. Almeida, P. Price, K. G. Ardlie, and G. W. Waterer. 2003b. Alleles carried at positions -819 and -592 of the IL10 promoter affect transcription following stimulation of peripheral blood cells with Streptococcus pneumoniae. *Immunogenetics* 55:629–32.

Temple, S. E., K. Y. Cheong, K. G. Ardlie, D. Sayer, and G. W. Waterer. 2004. The septic shock associated HSPA1B1267 polymorphism influences production of HSPA1A and HSPA1B. *Intensive Care Med* 30:1761–7.

Turner, D. M., D. M. Williams, D. Sankaran, M. Lazarus, P. J. Sinnott, and I. V. Hutchinson. 1997. An investigation of polymorphism in the interleukin-10 gene promoter. *Eur J Immunogenet* 24:1–8.

van der Pol, W. L., T. W. Huizinga, G. Vidarsson, M. W. van der Linden, M. D. Jansen, V. Keijsers, F. G. de Straat, N. A. Westerdaal, J. G. de Winkel, and R. G. Westendorp. 2001. Relevance of Fcgamma receptor and interleukin-10 polymorphisms for meningococcal disease. *J Infect Dis* 184:1548–55.

Walley, K., and J. Russell. 2007. Protein C -1641 AA is associated with decreased survival and more organ dysfunction in severe sepsis. *Crit Care Med* 35:12–17.

Watanabe, E., H. Hirasawa, S. Oda, K. Matsuda, M. Hatano, and T. Tokuhisa. 2005. Extremely high interleukin-6 blood levels and outcome in the critically ill are associated with tumor necrosis factor- and interleukin-1-related gene polymorphisms. *Crit Care Med* 33:89–97; discussion 242–3.

Waterer, G. W. 2007. Polymorphism studies in critical illness – we have to raise the bar. *Crit Care Med* 35:1424–5.

Waterer, G. W., M. W. Quasney, R. M. Cantor, and R. G. Wunderink. 2001. Septic shock and respiratory failure in community-acquired pneumonia have different TNF polymorphism associations. *Am J Respir Crit Care Med* 163:1599–604.

Waterer, G. W., L. ElBahlawan, M. W. Quasney, Q. Zhang, L. A. Kessler, and R. G. Wunderink. 2003. Heat shock protein 70-2+1267 AA homozygotes have an increased risk of septic shock in adults with community-acquired pneumonia. *Crit Care Med* 31:1367–72.

Wattanathum, A., S. Manocha, H. Groshaus, J. A. Russell, and K. R. Walley. 2005. Interleukin-10 haplotype associated with increased mortality in critically ill patients with sepsis from pneumonia but not in patients with extrapulmonary sepsis. *Chest* 128:1690–8.

Webb, K. E., J. F. Martin, J. Cotton, J. D. Erusalimsky, and S. E. Humphries. 2003. The 4830C > A polymorphism within intron 5 affects the pattern of alternative splicing occurring within exon 6 of the thrombopoietin gene. *Exp Hematol* 31:488–94.

Weiler, H., B. Kerlin, and M. C. Lytle. 2004. Factor V Leiden polymorphism modifies sepsis outcome: evidence from animal studies. *Crit Care Med* 32(5 Suppl):S233–8.

Westendorp, R. G., J. A. Langermans, T. W. Huizinga, A. H. Elouali, C. L. Verweij, D. I. Boomsma, and J. P. Vandenbroucke. 1997. Genetic influence on cytokine production and fatal meningococcal disease. *Lancet* 349(9046):170–3.

Yan, S. B., and D. R. Nelson. 2004. Effect of factor V Leiden polymorphism in severe sepsis and on treatment with recombinant human activated protein C. *Crit Care Med* 32(5 Suppl):S239–46.

Ye, S., F. R. Green, P. Y. Scarabin, V. Nicaud, L. Bara, S. J. Dawson, S. E. Humphries, A. Evans, G. Luc, J. P. Cambou, et al. 1995. The 4G/5G genetic polymorphism in the promoter of the plasminogen activator inhibitor-1 (PAI-1) gene is associated with differences in plasma PAI-1 activity but not with risk of myocardial infarction in the ECTIM study. Etude CasTemoins de I'nfarctus du Mycocarde. *Thromb Haemost* 74:837–41.

Ye, S. Q., B. A. Simon, J. P. Maloney, A. Zambelli-Weiner, L. Gao, A. Grant, R. B. Easley, B. J. McVerry, R. M. Tuder, T. Standiford, R. G. Brower, K. C. Barnes, and J. G. Garcia. 2005. Pre-B-cell colony-enhancing factor as a potential novel biomarker in acute lung injury. *Am J Respir Crit Care Med* 171:361–70.

Yee, A. M., S. C. Ng, R. E. Sobel, and J. E. Salmon. 1997. Fc gammaRIIA polymorphism as a risk factor for invasive pneumococcal infections in systemic lupus erythematosus. *Arthritis Rheum* 40:1180–2.

Yuan, F. F., M. Wong, N. Pererva, J. Keating, A. R. Davis, J. A. Bryant, and J. S. Sullivan. 2003. FcgammaRIIA polymorphisms in Streptococcus pneumoniae infection. *Immunol Cell Biol* 81:192–5.

Zhai, R., M. N. Gong, W. Zhou, T. B. Thompson, P. Kraft, L. Su, and D. C. Christiani. 2007. Genotypes and haplotypes of VEGF gene are associated with higher ARDS mortality and lower VEGF plasma levels. *Thorax* 62:718–22.

Chapter 4
Corticoids in Severe Pneumonia

Carlos Agustí, Oriol Sibila, and Antoni Torres

4.1 Introduction

Pneumonia is the most prevalent infectious respiratory disease. It entails high morbidity and mortality and large health system expenses.

Community-acquired pneumonia (CAP) is one of the five leading causes of death in the world. Approximately 20% of CAP patients require hospitalisation, 25% of which require intensive care unit (ICU) admission, and their mortality rate is of 40–50% (Alvarez-Lerma and Torres 2004).

Furthermore, 20–30% of patients under mechanical ventilation for at least 48 h in the ICU develop mechanical ventilation-associated pneumonia (VAP). Mortality attributable to VAP is also higher than 30%, being the leading cause of morbidity and mortality in patients with ICU-acquired nosocomial infections (ATS 2005).

Despite the progress in life support measures and in antimicrobial therapy, with the use of new antibiotics more efficient every time and with a broader spectrum, mortality of severe pneumonia has not varied during the last years (Lepper and Torres 1995; Heyland et al. 1999), suggesting that other factors are of crucial importance in the evolution of this respiratory infection.

One of the key factors determining the evolution of pneumonia is the host inflammatory response, increased excessively both in non-responding severe CAP and in VAP (Menéndez et al. 2004; Ioanas et al. 2004).

4.2 Inflammatory Response Associated with Pneumonia

It is well known that the arrival of pathogens to the alveolar space creates a complex inflammatory response with the action of several defence mechanisms and the production of several inflammatory mediators and acute-phase proteins (Sibille and Reynolds 1990).

This inflammatory response aims to control the progression of the infection and to destroy microorganisms, and consists of several pro-inflammatory (TNF-alpha, IL-1beta, IL-6 and IL-8) and anti-inflammatory (IL-10, IL-1RA, sTNFrp55 or sTNFrp75)

J. Rello, M.I. Restrepo (eds.) *Sepsis: New Strategies for Management.*
doi:10.1007/978-3-540-79001-3 © Springer-Verlag 2008

cytokines. Cytokines promote migration of defence cells – such as neutrophils, lymphocytes and platelets – through the circulatory system to inflammatory sites.

All this process will be beneficial as long as it is limited to the control of local infection. If this reaction is over-proportioned, several systemic consequences influence negatively the clinical evolution of the infection (Nelson et al. 1989).

Several studies have demonstrated that the inflammatory response can be reliably evaluated and that the determination of inflammatory mediators in serum and bronchoalveolar lavage (BAL) has diagnostic and prognostic value.

Studies have demonstrated an association between the increase of pro-inflammatory cytokines, such as IL-6 and TNF-alpha, and poor prognosis in sepsis (Martin et al. 1994). Studies concerning severe pneumonia showed that despite the local inflammatory response being initially compartmentalised (Dehoux et al. 1994), an increase of pro-inflammatory cytokines (IL-6, IL-8 and TNF-alpha) and anti-inflammatory cytokines (IL-10) in serum and in BAL was detected. These findings have also been related to poor prognosis of pneumonia (Montón et al. 1999a; Fernandez-Serrano et al. 2003).

In addition, a recent study of Yende et al. (2005) has demonstrated that patients with high levels of circulating cytokines in clinical stability (previous to infection) have a higher risk of suffering from community-acquired pneumonia, suggesting a crucial role of the inflammatory response in all the pathogenesis of this infection.

4.3   Glucocorticoids and Inflammatory Response

Due to the crucial importance of inflammatory response in the evolution of pneumonia, several anti-inflammatory treatments, with glucocorticoids (GC) being one of these, have been used in sepsis and in severe pneumonia.

GCs develop their action through their union to a specific intra-cytoplasmic receptor, the GC receptor (GR). After binding its ligand, the GR is activated and is translocated to the cell nucleus, where it binds DNA, producing an anti-inflammatory and immunosuppressive effect by two molecular mechanisms of action (see Table 4.1) (Rhen and Cidlowsly 2005): transrepression (or decrease in gene transcription of molecules with pro-inflammatory effect) and transactivation (or increase in gene transcription of molecules with anti-inflammatory effect.

GCs also provoke an anti-inflammatory effect by a third non-genomic mechanism of action: the activation of the endothelial nitric oxide synthetase (eNOS) which has a powerful effect on decrease in vascular inflammation.

In clinical practice, its usefulness seems demonstrated in several infections such as bacterial meningitis and pneumonia by *P. jiroveci* (Briel et al. 2005). In the field of sepsis, recent works by Keh et al. (2003) demonstrated that low dosages of hydrocortisone achieved quick haemodynamic stabilisation in patients with septic shock. This study verified that hydrocortisone attenuates the inflammatory and anti-inflammatory response, but does not have a negative effect on the phagocyte function of macrophages and monocytes.

Table 4.1 Effect of glucocorticoids in gene transcription

Decrease of gene transcription (transrepression)
- Cytokines (IL-1, IL-2, IL-3, IL-4, IL-5, IL-6, IL-8, IL-11, IL-13, tumoral necrosis factor alpha, granulocytes and macrophages colonies stimulating factors)
- Chemokines (RANTES, eotoxin, macrophage inflammatory protein 1 alpha (MIP-1α), monocytes 1 and 3 chemotactic proteins)
- Enzymes (inducible nitric oxide synthetase, cyclooxygenase 2, cytoplasmic phospholipase A2)
- Adhesion molecules (intracellular adhesion molecule 1, vascular cells adhesion molecule 1)
- Receptors (IL-2 receptor, tachikinin 1 (NK-1))

Increase of gene transcription (transactivation)
- Lipocortin 1
- Receptors β2
- SLPI (serum leukoprotease inhibitor)
- Clear cells protein (CC10, phospholipase A2 inhibitor)
- Antagonist of the IL-1 receptor
- Inhibitor of the nuclear factor kappa B
- IL-10

IL interleukin

4.4 Role of Glucocorticoids in Severe Pneumonia

The first studies conducted in patients with sepsis and pneumonia suggested a rapid improvement of symptoms in patients receiving GC, although effects in mortality were not evidenced, and some cases were associated with a higher number of side effects and to a poorer prognosis once the steroid treatment was suspended (Lefering and Neugbauer 1995). These contradictory findings were mostly due to the lack of knowledge on the role of the inflammatory response in the prognosis of this disease and its possible therapeutic modulation by GC.

A pilot work by Montón et al. in patients with severe pneumonia requiring mechanical ventilation (Montón et al. 1999) detected the possible immunosuppressive effect of GC in pneumonia, since the authors observed a decrease in pro-inflammatory cytokines, such as IL-6 and TNF-alpha, both in serum and in bronchoalveolar lavage of patients who received GC as co-adjuvant treatment (in most cases as a bronchodilator treatment associated with the antibiotic treatment). Furthermore, in the group of patients receiving GC treatment, a tendency to lower mortality was observed, although the population of the study was represented by only 20 patients.

The relationship between the intensity of the inflammatory response in severe pneumonia, GC dosage and the prognosis of this disease was subsequently studied by Agustí et al. (2003). In this study, the authors assessed the inflammatory response in bronchoalveolar lavage and in serum of patients with severe pneumonia who received GC treatment for long periods (>30 days). Results were compared to those from a group of patients with severe pneumonia without GC treatment and another group of patients with pneumonia and GC treatment, in most of the cases as a bronchodilator treatment, for a short period of time (9 ± 7 days).

These authors observed that the local inflammatory response (in BAL) and systemic inflammatory response (in serum), measured by such relevant cytokines as IL-6 or TNF-alpha, was markedly diminished in patients who received GC for long periods of time compared to patients who had not received such treatment. Furthermore, acute administration of GC had an intermediate effect in the suppression of the inflammatory response.

Mortality in the group of patients with severe pneumonia and prolonged corticoid treatment was similar to mortality of patients who did not receive GC treatment. Interestingly, patients who received GC treatment for short periods of time and showing an attenuated inflammatory response had, on the contrary, a tendency to lower mortality.

These results suggested that deep attenuation of the inflammatory response by prolonged corticoid treatment can be as harmful as an exaggerated inflammatory response, but its "moderated" attenuation by a short corticoid treatment can be beneficial for the modulation of the inflammatory response and for the prognosis of the disease.

In another work by Ioanas et al. (2004), in a series of patients with ICU-acquired pneumonia requiring mechanical ventilation, the authors found that high levels of IL-6 and IL-8 at the time of diagnosis and IL-6 levels on day 3 were the only factors related to the lack of response to empiric antibiotic treatment, suggesting again that the potential inflammatory response modulation could be beneficial also in this subgroup of patients. Furthermore, in the multivariate analysis of the several factors that could be related to the lack of response to treatment, the authors found that the concomitant administration of GC was a protective factor (OR 0.21).

In a recent work by Sibila and collaborators (2006) in an experimental model of severe pneumonia in ventilated pigs, in which the effect of GCs was studied by comparing three groups of animals with severe pneumonia induced by *Pseudomonas aeruginosa* (without treatment, with antibiotic treatment and with antibiotic treatment + GC), the authors evidenced that pigs treated with antibiotics + GC experimented, after 96h of pneumonia onset, a decrease in the local inflammatory response compared to other groups.

Furthermore, animals treated with antibiotics and steroids presented lower bacterial count both in bronchoalveolar lavage and in pulmonary tissue obtained in the end of the 96-h study, a finding that was related to a clear tendency to suffer from less severe lesions, as revealed by the histopathological study.

Finally, animals treated with steroids also showed an improvement in pulmonary mechanics (measured by means of static compliance) compared with the rest of the group.

Although all these findings seem to point to the beneficial effect of the steroid treatment in severe pneumonia, a confirmation of these potential benefits is needed in randomised and controlled clinical trials.

According to these premises, Confalonieri and collaborators (Confalonieri et al. 2005) assessed the efficiency and safety of the administration of a continuous infusion of hydrocortisone in a double-blind, randomised, placebo-controlled trial including 46 patients with severe CAP requiring ICU admission.

An intravenous bolus of hydrocortisone, in a dose of 200 mg followed by a perfusion of 10 mg/h during 7 days, was given to 23 patients. These authors demonstrated a mortality reduction in the group treated with hydrocortisone (0% vs. 30%), a better modulation of systemic inflammatory response (determined by serum C-reactive protein) and a significant improvement in the main clinical endpoints, such as thorax X-ray, MODS severity scale, PaO2/FiO2 coefficient and ICU and hospital stay.

These results show that the modulation of systemic inflammation with early administration of GC can improve the evolution of community-acquired pneumonia and prevent possible complications from a secondary sepsis, thus improving mortality.

4.5   Pending Questions

Before being able to generalise the use of GC in patients afflicted with severe pneumonia, some questions must be specified.

Firstly, the spectacular results of the study by Confalonieri et al. (2005) must be confirmed by studies including a higher number of patients, with no differences between the two groups of the study. In the aforementioned work, the group receiving GC presented at the beginning of the study a significantly higher systemic inflammation level (measured by the blood C-reactive protein) than the group that did not receive corticoid treatment.

Another important aspect is the moment of suppression of the steroid treatment. An early suspension of GC can be potentially dangerous if pro-inflammatory cytokines increase again and their receptors continue being suppressed. Studies conducted in patients with septic shock have demonstrated that hydrocortisone infusion produces significant decrease in the circulating levels of proteins depending on the nuclear factor kappa B transcription (NF-κB), such as phospholipase A2, IL-6, IL-8 and soluble E-selectin. On the one hand, the suppression of the treatment provokes a rebound effect in most of these mediators, which highlights the short anti-inflammatory action of hydrocortisone and the need for administering a prolonged treatment to achieve a durable anti-inflammatory effect (Briegel et al. 1994). On the other hand, the prolonged use of corticoids can entail a suppression of the innate immune function since it alters the phagocyte action of macrophages and alveolar granulocytes, which can facilitate the acquisition of very severe bacterial infections and of opportunist microbes (Meersseman et al. 2004). Consequently, studies are needed to determine the duration of treatment with a special emphasis of the initial dosage, the maintenance time and the type of suspension.

Finally, other questions without an answer are related to the appropriate type of glucocorticoid for this treatment (hydrocortisone, methylprednisolone), and to a better study of the suprarenal function in patients with severe pneumonia and its potential modulation by GC (Annane et al. 2002).

4.6 Conclusions

Current information suggests that treatment with low dosages of GC in severe pneumonia is able to modulate (or diminish) the inflammatory response associated with pneumonia and improve the prognosis of this disease, mainly in cases where an increased host inflammatory response is demonstrated.

Scientific evidence is still scarce, and ample randomised and controlled clinical trials are needed to claim the aforementioned affirmation. Furthermore, it is of uppermost importance to design studies not only to get a better understanding of the effect of GC in severe pneumonia, but also to determine the type of GC, the dosage to administer and the duration of the treatment.

References

Agustí C, Rañó A, Filella X, et al. Pulmonary infiltrates in patients receiving long-term glucocorticoid treatment. Etiology, prognostic factors and associated inflammatory response. Chest 2003; 123: 488–498.

Alvarez-Lerma F, Torres A. Severe community-acquired pneumonia. Curr Opin Crit Care 2004; 10: 369–374.

American Thoracic Society. Guidelines for the management of adults with hospital-acquired pneumonia, ventilator-associated pneumonia and healthcare-associated pneumonia. Am J Respir Crit Care Med 2005; 171: 388–416.

Annane D, Sébille V, Charpentier C, et al. Effect of treatment with low doses of hydrocortisone and fludrocortisone on mortality in patients with septic shock. JAMA 2002; 288: 862–871.

Briegel J, Kellermann W, Forst H, et al. Low-dose hydrocortisone infusion attenuates the systemic inflammatory response syndrome. Clin Invest 1994; 72: 782–787.

Briel M, Boscacci R, Furrer H, et al. Adjunctive corticoesteroids for Pneumocysti jiroveci pneumonia in patients with HIV infection: a meta-analysis of randomized controlled trials. BMC Infect Dis 2005; 5: 101.

Confalonieri R, Rubino G, Carbone A, et al. Hydrocortisone infusion for severe community-acquired pneumonia: a preliminary randomised study. Am J Respir Crit Care Med 2005; 171: 242–248.

Dehoux MS, Boutten A, Ostinelli J, et al. Compartmentalized cytokine production within the human lung in unilateral pneumonia. Am J Respir Crit Care Med 1994; 150: 710–716.

Fernandez-Serrano S, Dorca J, Coromines M, et al. Molecular inflammatory response measured in blood of patients with severe community-acquired pneumonia. Clin Diagn Lab Immunol 2003; 10: 813–820.

Heyland DK, Cook DJ, Griffith L, et al. The attributable morbidity and mortality of ventilator-associated pneumonia in the critically ill patient. Am J Respir Crit Care Med 1999; 159: 1249–1256.

Ioanas M, Ferrer M, Cavalcanti M, et al. Causes and predictors of nonresponse to treatment of ICU-acquired pneumonia. Crit Care Med 2004; 32: 938–945.

Keh D, Boenhke T, Weber-Cartens S, et al. Immunologic and hemodynamic effects of "low-dose" hydrocortisone in septic shock. A double blind, randomised, placebo-controlled, crossover study. Am J Respir Crit Care Med 2003; 167: 512–520.

Leeper KV, Torres A. Community-acquired pneumonia in the intensive care unit. Clin Chest Med 1995; 16: 155–171.

Lefering R, Neugebauer EM. Steroid controversy in sepsis and septic shock: a meta-analysis. Crit Care Med 1995; 23: 1294–1303.

Martin C, Sauzx P, Mege JL, et al. Prognostic value of serum cytokines in septic shock. Intensive Care Med 1994; 20: 272–277.

Meersseman W, Vandecasteele SJ, Wilmer A, et al. Invasive aspergillosis in critically ill patients without malignancies. Am J Respir Crit Care Med 2004; 170: 621–625.

Menéndez R, Torres A, Rodriguez de Castro F, et al. Predictive factors of clinical stability in community-acquired pneumonia. Thorax 2004; 59: 960–965.

Montón C, Ewig S, Torres A, et al. Role of glucocorticoids on inflammatory response in nonimmunosuppressed patients with pneumonia: a pilot study. Eur Respir J 1999a; 14: 218–220.

Montón C, Torres A, el-Ebiary M, et al. Cytokine expression in severe pneumonia: a bronchoalveolar study. Crit Care Med 1999b; 27: 1745–1753.

Nelson S, Bagby GJ, Bainton BG, et al. Compartimentalization of intraalveolar and systemic lipopolysaccharide-induced tumor necrosis factor and the pulmonary inflammatory response. J Infect Dis 1989; 159: 189–194.

Rhen T, Cidlowsky JA. Antiinflammatory action of glucocorticoids – new mechanisms for old drugs. N Engl J Med 2005; 353: 1711–1723.

Sibila O, Luna CM, Agustí C, et al. Effect of corticoesteroids in an animal model of ventilator-associated pneumonia. Am J Respir Crit Care Med 2006; 3: A21.

Sibille Y, Reynolds HY. Macrophages and polymorphonuclear neutrophils in lung defense and injury. Am Rev Respir Dis 1990; 141: 471–501.

Yende S, Tuomanen EI, Wunderink RG, et al. Pre-infection systemic inflammatory markers and risk of hospitalisation due to pneumonia. Am J Respir Crit Care Med 2005; 172: 535–541.

Chapter 5
Aging, Inflammation, and Pneumococcal Disease

Angela J. Rodriguez and Carlos J. Orihuela

5.1 Introduction

Streptococcus pneumoniae (the pneumococcus) is the leading cause of community-acquired pneumonia (CAP) and otitis media, and a primary cause of bacteremia and meningitis (Pneumococcal vaccines 1999). As with most infectious diseases, the poorest nations experience the greatest burden of disease. This can be attributed to reduced vaccine use, decreased standards of living, and limited access to supportive critical care (Dopazo et al. 2001; Robinson et al. 2001). Worldwide, the incidence of invasive pneumococcal disease (IPD) is greatest in children. However, death, as a result of infection, primarily occurs in the elderly (>65 years of age) (Atkinson et al. 2007; Lexau et al. 2005). The World Health Organization (WHO) estimates that pneumococcal disease is responsible for 1.6 million deaths annually (Pneumococcal vaccines 1999).

Pneumococcal disease in the elderly is characterized by its rapid onset, severity, and high case-fatality rate; in the United States, the mortality rate for the elderly with pneumococcal pneumonia is 13–23%, compared to 5–7% in the general population. Likewise, case-fatality rates for the elderly with pneumococcal bacteremia and meningitis are 60% and 80%, respectively; in contrast, they are 20% and 30% for the general population (Atkinson et al. 2007). Risk factors for IPD include advanced age, alcoholism, bronchial asthma, immunosuppression, lung disease, heart disease, asplenia, diabetes, and institutionalization (Loeb 2004; Mufson 1999). It is of note that the majority of the elderly have one or more underlying medical conditions that puts them at increased risk for IPD (Robinson et al. 2001). Moreover, the elderly experience age-related changes in immune function that increase their susceptibility to infection.

5.1.1 Clinical Presentation

Clinical presentation of pneumonia in healthy adults includes fatigue, fever, chills, anorexia, sweats, myalgia, pleuritic chest pain, and cough with purulent sputum production (Johnson 2000; Koivula 1994). In the elderly, there are often fewer

J. Rello, M.I. Restrepo (eds.) *Sepsis: New Strategies for Management.*
doi:10.1007/978-3-540-79001-3 © Springer-Verlag 2008

symptoms including a lack of fever or cough (Granton and Grossman 1993). Notably, absence of fever has been associated with a poor prognosis. Elderly patients with pneumonia often present with neurological symptoms, in particular an altered mental state. By and large it is dependent on the physician to recognize that the lack of overt clinical signs does not rule out the possibility of pneumonia in the elderly and that diagnosis of pneumonia is dependent on a thorough pulmonary lung exam and most importantly, visualization by chest X-ray of lobar involvement.

It is beyond the scope of this review to detail clinical management of pneumococcal pneumonia, bacteremia, or sepsis. However, several studies have documented that antibiotic therapy within the first 8 h of hospitalization was associated with decreased 30-day mortality rates (Loeb 2004; Niederman et al. 2001). Currently, the American Thoracic Society guidelines for treatment of pneumonia include administration of a second-generation cephalosporin with a macrolide, sulfamethoxazole-trimethoprim, or β-lactam with a macrolide if a susceptible strain is found (Niederman et al. 2001).

5.1.2 Vaccines

Immunity against pneumococcal disease is mediated by antibodies against the capsular serotype involved. At this time, only one vaccine, Pneumovax® 23 (Merck & Co. Inc.), is licensed by the United States Food and Drug Administration for use in adults against *S. pneumoniae*. Pneumovax® 23 is composed of capsular polysaccharide (CPS) from the 23 most common serotypes and has an overall protective efficacy of 55–70% against bacteremia and meningitis (Pneumococcal vaccines 1999; Shapiro et al. 1991). Unfortunately, Pneumovax® 23 does not protect against nonbacteremic disease (i.e., pneumonia without bloodstream infection) (French et al. 2000; Whitney et al. 2003). This is a major concern, as *S. pneumoniae* is the most frequent cause of CAP, and CAP is most severe in the elderly (Lexau et al. 2005; Gutierrez et al. 2006; Janssens 2005). In addition, the elderly do not produce a robust response to the vaccine as evidenced by a lack of protective antibody to the polysaccharide capsule (Bruyn and Van Furth 1991; Regev-Yochay et al. 2004). Currently, the United States Centers for Disease Control and Prevention recommends vaccination of all high-risk groups, and revaccination of the elderly every 5 years.

Children in the United States are vaccinated with a conjugate vaccine composed of CPS linked to the diphtheria toxoid (Prevnar®; Wyeth Inc.). Use of Prevnar® has not only led to a decrease in the incidence of IPD among children, but also to decreased nasopharyngeal colonization of the serotypes included in the vaccine (Whitney et al. 2003; McBean et al. 2006). Decreased carriage rates have in turn led to improved "herd immunity" and a reduction in incidence of IPD in the elderly. From 1998 to 2003, the incidence of invasive disease among the elderly has decreased by 18% (McBean et al. 2006).

Vaccination is the only proven method shown to reduce IPD. Unfortunately, protein conjugation is costly and imposes steric hindrances that limit the numbers of capsule types that can be included in a vaccine formulation. Prevnar® is composed of CPS from seven of the >90 known serotypes (Pneumococcal vaccines 1999; MMWR Recomm Rep 2000). Thus, children vaccinated with Prevnar® remain colonized and are susceptible to nonvaccine serotypes. Due to the limited number of serotypes included in Prevnar®, vaccine efficacy is reduced in countries where nonvaccine serotypes are more frequently the cause of disease; for example, Prevnar® protects against only 58% of the serotypes that cause invasive disease in Latin America (Sniadack et al. 1995). Studies are currently being conducted on protein conjugate vaccines composed of CPS from 9 and 11 serotypes. These would improve coverage in developing countries. However, cost of the vaccine and the implementations of policies that ensure its use remain daunting obstacles not only in South American countries but also in most of the world.

5.2 Bacterial Pathogenesis

5.2.1 Microbiology

S. pneumoniae is a gram-positive diplococcus that grows in pairs or short chains and is catalase negative. Most laboratories grow the bacteria on tryptic soy agar supplemented with blood in 5% CO_2. These culture conditions are preferred as blood contains a high level of catalase and Streptococcus spp. are facultative anaerobes. Currently, pneumococci are identified in a microbiology laboratory by: α-hemolysis on blood agar plates, catalase negativity, susceptibility to optochin, and solubility to bile salts. Pneumococci are also now identified by detecting ribosomal RNA that is specific to the pneumococcus.

5.2.2 Inflammation Resulting from Infection

Solely a human pathogen, the pneumococcus colonizes the nasopharynx and is spread among humans by aerosol droplets. IPD results from the spread of the pneumococcus from the nasopharynx to the lungs, blood stream, and central nervous system. While attack rates are generally low, such a large number of individuals are colonized that the resulting morbidity and mortality associated with the pneumococcus is tremendous. Pneumococcal disease is characterized by an intense inflammatory response that, in the lungs, results in consolidation of the infected alveoli and the affected lobe. Infected lung tissue progresses through stages of engorgement during which capillaries and epithelial cells become inflamed; fluid, erythrocytes and neutrophils accumulate in the alveoli; and a fibrin mesh develops (red hepatization). Subsequently, the lungs darken (gray hepatization) as leukocytes enter the lesion and the bacteria are engulfed by neutrophils and macrophages.

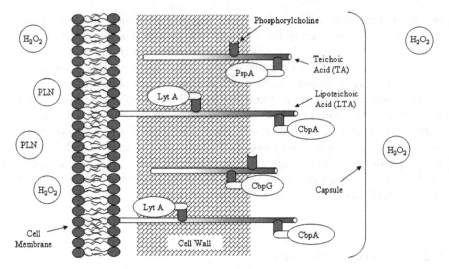

Fig. 5.1 Representation of *S. pneumoniae* cell membrane, cell wall and capsule. Within the bacteria is the toxin pneumolysin (PLN), which is released along with cell wall fragments following lysis of the bacteria. Cell lysis can be the result of cell death or autolysis triggered by cell-wall-acting antimicrobials such as β-lactams. The cell wall consists of peptidoglycan and is covalently linked to teichoic acid (TA). Lipotechoic acid (LTA) extends from the cell membrane through the cell wall. Both TA and LTA contain phosphorylcholine residues that bind to PAFr and serve as anchors to a family of proteins known as choline-binding proteins: choline-binding protein A (CbpA) is an adhesin and mediates attachment to pIgR. Choline-binding protein G (CbpG) is a protease required for replication to high titer in the blood. Pneumococcal surface protein A (PspA) inhibits complement deposition by binding to factor H. Finally, the murein hydrolyse, autolysin (LytA), is also a choline-binding protein. During growth, the bacteria release hydrogen peroxide. This contributes to tissue damage caused by the bacteria

Resolution continues for several days as capsule-specific antibodies provide efficient opsonization and inflammatory mediators dissipate (Tuomanen 2004).

Pneumococcal cell wall, pneumolysin, and hydrogen peroxide are the primary virulence determinants that mediate the inflammation and cytotoxicity that is observed in the lungs (see Fig. 5.1) (Berry and Paton 2000; Canvin et al. 1995). Intratracheal challenge of mice with purified pneumolysin or cell wall products is sufficient to cause edema and the influx of neutrophils that result in pneumonia (Regew-Yochay et al. 2004; Tuomanen et al. 1987). Multiple studies demonstrate that deletion of the genes that encode autolysin (LytA), the bacteria cell wall hydrolase, pneumolysin (Pln), a pore-forming toxin, or pyruvate oxidase, the enzyme that produces hydrogen peroxide, results in attenuated bacteria that are unable to survive in the lungs (Regew-Yochay et al. 2004; Berry and Paton 2000; Berry et al. 1992; Orihuela et al. 2004). These findings suggest that the ability of the pneumococcus to cause inflammation is not incidental but a requirement for its survival in vivo. Importantly, because the pneumococcus is encapsulated, phagocytosis is limited until sufficient capsule-specific antibodies are present. Prior to this, the thick peptidoglycan cell wall layer protects the bacteria from complement-mediated killing.

Inflammation is requisite for clearance of the bacteria. Proinflammatory mediators such as activated complement (activated complement protein C3a, C5a), tumor necrosis factor alpha (TNFα), interleukin (IL)-1, and macrophage inflammatory protein 2 (MIP-2) contribute to the influx of neutrophils (PMNs) and macrophages that are the effector cells in the host defense against pneumococcal pneumonia (Regev-Yochay et al. 2004; Kadioglu et al. 2000). In mice, PMNs appear in the lungs 2–4 h after challenge and increase in number up to 48 h after infection (Dallaire et al. 2001). Not surprisingly, excessive inflammation is detrimental. Continued production of inflammatory mediators and PMN recruitment has been associated with death following intranasal and intratracheal challenge of mice with *S. pneumoniae*. Likewise, studies have documented an association between survival and an earlier disappearance of lung PMNs (Dallaire et al. 2001; Burns et al. 2005). Most recently, Marks et al. have shown that mice depleted of neutrophils and challenged with a serotype 8 isolate of *S. pneumoniae* had less lung damage, longer survival, and less lung apoptosis than control mice (Marks et al. 2007). Thus, an excessive immune response, where the host defense causes tissue damage and lung consolidation, contributes to pneumococcal-associated mortality.

5.2.3 Toll-Like Receptors (TLRs) Detect Microorganisms and Initiate the Innate Host Defense

TLRs are a family of surface receptors that recognize pathogen-associated molecular patterns (i.e., structural components) present in bacteria, viruses and fungi. Binding of ligands to TLRs initiates an intracellular signaling cascade through cytoplasmic intermediates such as TIR, Myd88, and IRAK that ultimately results in NFkB activation and production of proinflammatory cytokines. TLRs are sensors that activate the innate immune system. Thus, deficiencies in TLR functions result in diminished cytokine production and an increased susceptibility to infection (Akira and Sato 2003; Takeda et al. 2003). Pertinent to this review, TLR-2 and TLR-4 are the sensors responsible for the detection of *S. pneumoniae* and are expressed on a wide variety of cell types including mucosal epithelial cells and alveolar macrophages (Armstrong et al. 2004; Saito et al. 2005).

Peptidoglycan (PGN) is the primary constituent of bacterial cell wall, composed of alternating *N*-acetylglucosamine and *N*-acetylmuramic acid residues cross-linked by short peptides. Instilled peptidoglycan can reproduce most of the clinical manifestations of bacterial infections including fever, inflammation, and septic shock. Most of these effects are the result of cytokines that are released from macrophages (Fournier and Philpott 2005; Pichichero et al. 2005). It is now known that peptidoglycan initiates inflammation through its activation of TLR-2. Peptidoglycan binds to lipopolysaccharide-binding protein (LBP) (Weber et al. 2003), which in turn binds to CD14 (Dziarski et al. 1998, 2000; Gupta et al. 1996, 1999). Binding of LBP:peptidoglycan to CD14 induces physical proximity of the CD14:LBP:

peptidoglycan complex with TLR-2/TLR-1 and formation of the TLR-2 signaling complex (Becker et al. 2002; Manukyan et al. 2005).

Pneumolysin is also released by *S. pneumoniae* during bacteria lysis. Pneumolysin binds to cholesterol on the host cell membrane, and at high concentrations oligomerizes and forms lytic pores (Edwards 2004). Low concentrations of pneumolysin have been shown to have multiple effects including stimulating the production of TNFα and IL-1β by human mononuclear phagocytes (Houldsworth et al. 1994), inducing nitric oxide (NO) production from macrophages (Braun et al. 2002), and phosphorylation of p38 MAPK in epithelial cells (Ratner et al. 2005). Evidence now indicates that pneumolysin binds to TLR-4 (Malley et al. 2003). Srivastava et al. (2005) found that macrophages from wild-type mice were significantly more prone to pneumolysin-induced apoptosis than cells from TLR-4-defective mice and pretreatment of epithelial cells with TLR-4 antagonist reduced pneumolysin-mediated apoptosis in wild-type cells (Srivastava et al. 2005). Together, pneumolysin and pneumococcal cell wall act synergistically to activate host cells. In contrast, macrophages from TLR-4-deficient mice were hyporesponsive to pneumolysin and the combination of pneumolysin with cell wall (Srivastava et al. 2005; Malley et al. 2003).

5.3 Inflammation Increases Susceptibility to IPD

The process of inflammation is normally a protective mechanism that is employed by the host to destroy, dilute, or wall off infecting agents. During the past 25 years it has also become evident that aging is associated with chronic low-grade inflammation (Sarkar and Fisher 2006). Studies by multiple investigators have shown that individuals >65 years experience higher levels of proinflammatory cytokines in blood and tissues than healthy young adults Bruunsgaard et al. 2001; Ershler 1993; Paolisso et al. 1998). Age-associated inflammation (AAI) can be the result of multiple factors including chronic underlying diseases, obesity, diabetes, and the aging process itself, a side effect of cellular senescence, and an increased production of reactive oxygen species (Krabbe et al. 2004; Bruunsgaard et al. 1999).

In the lungs, studies by Meyer et al. have shown that the healthy elderly have increased numbers of neutrophils, IL-6, and immunoglobulin in bronchoalveolar lavage when compared to younger subjects (Meyer et al. 1996). Likewise, Meyer et al. observed an increased ratio of CD4+ cells to CD8+ cells (Meyer and Soergel 1999). Examination of tissues from aged rodents supports the notion of AAI and demonstrates that aged mice have higher levels of NFkB activation in the brain, lungs, liver, spleen, and lymphoid tissues (Spencer et al. 1997). Briefly, NFkB serves as the central transcription factor responsible for inflammation (Sarkar and Fisher 2006; Xiao and Ghosh 2005). Tissue samples from aged mice also express higher levels of TNF, IL-6, IL-12, and COX-2 when compared to young adult mice (Spencer et al. 1997). These findings suggest that even when there are no apparent signs of infection or disease, increased levels of inflammation are present in the elderly.

5.3.1 Individuals with Increased Inflammation Have More Frequent and Severe IPD

Increased inflammation is pertinent to pneumococcal disease, as elevated levels of proinflammatory cytokines in the blood have been correlated with an increased incidence of pneumococcal pneumonia and heightened severity of infection. For example, Yende et al. (2005) document that elevated levels of IL-6 and TNFα in the blood are associated with increased risk for CAP. Individuals with the highest levels of TNFα and IL-6 in serum experienced a 1.8- to 2.8-fold increase in the incidence of CAP over a 6.5-year period (upper tertile vs. lower tertile), a finding that was determined to be independent of coexisting medical condition, smoking status, and steroid use. Likewise, studies by Glynn et al. (1999) and Antunes et al. (2002) found that IL-6 correlated best with both disease-specific and generic severity scores for pneumonia. Thus inflammation links age with risk for IPD.

5.3.2 S. pneumoniae Adhesion and Invasion is Dependent on Inflammation

S. pneumoniae attachment and invasion is dependent on activation of NFkB and cellular inflammation. While attachment of the pneumococcus is initially mediated by loose interactions with glycoconjugates (Cundell and Tuomanen 1994), invasion does not occur until the cells become activated (i.e., NFkB is translocated into the nucleus) and the cell expresses the NFkB-regulated host proteins polymeric immunoglobulin receptor (pIgR) and platelet-activating factor receptor (PAFr) to which the pneumococcus binds to (Cundell et al. 1995; Zhang et al. 2000). In healthy adults, cell activation occurs during infection following contact with bacterial components such as peptidoglycan and pneumolysin. In contrast, in the elderly, elevated pIgR and PAFr levels are already present in the lungs, the result of age-associated inflammation or proinflammatory cytokines in blood as a result of underlying disease (see Fig. 5.2 and 5.3). Once the cell is activated, bacterial adherence is increased and invasion is mediated by the bacterial protein choline-binding protein A (CbpA) and phosphorylcholine (ChoP) on the cell wall. CbpA binds to pIgR on epithelial cells, while ChoP binds to PAFr on epithelial and endothelial cells. In general, the pneumococcus is a low-efficiency invader with ~0.2% of the inoculum invading cells (Cundell et al. 1995); nonetheless, invasion is a critical step in the development of IPD and is the mechanism by which the bacterium enters the central nervous system (Orihuela et al. 2004).

5.3.3 pIgR-Mediated Invasion

In the respiratory tract, pneumococcal adherence and invasion is mediated by the bacterial protein CbpA (Orihuela et al. 2004; Zhang et al. 2000). CbpA binds to

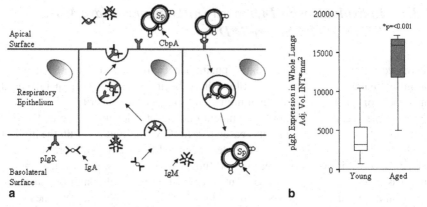

Fig. 5.2 (**a**) pIgR-mediated transport of *S. pneumoniae*. Secretory IgA is the first line of the specific immune defense that is encountered by bacteria invading the lungs. Epithelial cells in the respiratory tract transport polymeric IgA from the basolateral surface to the lumen through a series of vacuoles resulting in the presence of a pIgR/antibody complex on the apical surface. Cleavage of this complex permits the release of the antibody and a portion of the receptor that remains attached to the antibody (secretory component); secretory component protects the antibody from proteolytic degradation. Importantly, unoccupied pIgR on the apical surface is recycled, and returns to the basolateral surface for subsequent attachment to immunoglobulin. *S. pneumoniae* co-opts this system by binding to unoccupied pIgR on the apical surface through CbpA and is translocated through the cell during receptor recycling. (**b**) Elevated levels of pIgR in the lungs of aged mice vs. young. Box plot demonstrating increased expression of pIgR in the lungs of aged (19-month old, $n = 6$) vs. young (4-month old, $n = 6$) female Balb/cBy mice (unpublished finding). Whole lungs were homogenized and levels of pIgR were determined by measuring band intensity on immunoblots. *Box* indicates 25–75% percentile, *horizontal bar* indicates average, *inner and outer fence* indicate lowest and highest value

the pIgR machinery and allows translocation of the bacteria to the basolateral surface (see Fig. 5.2) (Kaetzel 2001). Zhang et al. have demonstrated that wild-type, but not CbpA-deficient *S. pneumoniae* adhere to pIgR and are transported to the basolateral surface during receptor recycling (Zhang et al. 2000). This interaction is inhibited by the addition of antibodies to CbpA, antibodies to secretory component (SC), and purified SC, all of which reduce pneumococcal adhesion and invasion. Furthermore, mice deficient in pIgR, and mice deficient in the protein tyrosine kinase p62[yes], which is required for pIgR transcytosis, demonstrate decreased nasopharyngeal colonization and a delayed onset of bacteremia relative to wild type (Luton et al. 1999). Finally, Rosenow et al. demonstrate that CbpA deficient bacteria colonize the nasopharynx at a 100-fold lower efficiency than wild-type bacteria (Rosenow et al. 1997).

Importantly, pIgR expression is enhanced following NFkB activation and has been observed to be elevated in the lungs of aged mice (see Fig. 5.2b). Zhang et al.

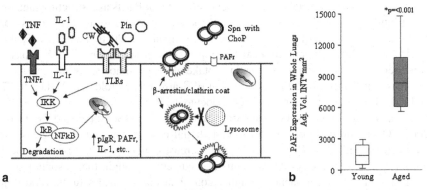

Fig. 5.3 (a) Platelet-activating factor receptor (PAFr) and NFkB activation. NFkB activation can be the result of various stimuli such as binding of peptidoglycan (CW) and pneumolysin (Pln) to TLRs and cell exposure to proinflammatory cytokines such as TNF and IL-1. Binding of ligands to their receptors initiates a cell-signaling cascade (not shown) which results in IkB kinase (IKK) activation. IKK then phosphorylates inhibitor kB (IkB) which leads to its dissociation from nuclear-factor kappa B (NFkB). NFkB is then able to enter the nucleus and serve as a transcriptional activator to numerous pro- and anti-inflammatory mediators including PAFr. PAFr on the cell surface binds to phosphorylcholine (ChoP), a component of teichoic and lipoteichoic acid residues on the bacteria. This activates ERK kinases leading to the formation of clathrin-coated vesicles that mediate endocytosis and passage of pneumococci through the cell. (b) Elevated levels of PAFr in the lungs of aged mice vs. young. *Box plot* demonstrating increased expression of PAFr in the lungs of aged (19-month old, $n = 6$) vs. young (4-month old, $n = 6$) female Balb/cBy mice (unpublished finding). Whole lungs were homogenized and levels of PAFr were determined by measuring band intensity on immunoblots. *Box* indicates 25–75% percentile, *horizontal bar* indicates average, *inner* and *outer fence* indicate lowest and highest value

have demonstrated that treatment of Detroit cells, a nasopharyngeal cell line, for 12 h with IFNγ increased bacterial adhesion and invasion. Furthermore, Bruno and Kaetzel demonstrate that chronic exposure (2 weeks) of HT-29 cell to TNFα resulted in a 7- to 20-fold increase in the amount of pIgR transcribed (Bruno and Kaetzel 2005). Thus, inflammation increases pIgR expression, which in turn increases pneumococcal attachment and invasion, a finding that explains how AAI may facilitate the development of IPD.

5.3.4 PAFr-Mediated Invasion

S. pneumoniae also attaches to PAFr, the chemokine receptor for platelet-activating factor (Cundell et al. 1995; Zhang et al. 2000). PAFr binding is mediated by phosphorylcholine (ChoP), which is present on the bacterial cell wall and lipoteichoic residues that extend from the cell membrane (see Fig. 5.1). Phosphorylcholine is a structural component of PAF and it is believed that ChoP acts as a structural analog when binding to PAFr. Unlike PAF, pneumococcus binding to the PAFr does not result in the activation of a G-protein-mediated signal transduction pathway (Radin et al. 2005). Rather, pneumococcal binding results in activation of ERK kinases consistent with activation by β-arrestin. Uptake of the pneumococcus into a vacuole involves clatherin followed by recruitment of β-arrestin scaffold, Rab5, then Rab7 and Rab11. Rab 5 is involved in early endocytosis, Rab 7 is found in the late endosome, and Rab 11 is responsible for vacuole recycling (Seachrist and Ferguson 2003). Overexpression of arrestin in endothelial cells enhances colocalization of the bacteria with Rab 7 and Rab 11 and increases survival of the pneumococci normally killed by the lysozyme. Thus it is currently thought that association of β-arrestin with the PAFr vacuole complex contributes to the successful translocation of the bacteria away from the lysozyme (Radin et al. 2005). Of note, PAFr-mediated invasion of endothelial cells requires CbpA, although CbpA does not bind PAFr, suggesting the presence of a second stabilizing ligand (Hoskins et al. 2001).

It is well documented that *S. pneumoniae* preferentially binds to cells treated with proinflammatory cytokines. Like pIgR, PAFr is regulated by NFkB (Cundell et al. 1995; Zhang et al. 2000) and is produced de novo following exposure of cells to proinflammatory cytokines, cell wall components, and reactive oxygen species (Silverman et al. 2001). Unlike pIgR, PAFr is expressed ubiquitously on both epithelial and endothelial cells. Binding of bacteria to PAFr is thought to be a principal mechanism by which the bacteria enter the bloodstream and the sole mechanism as to how bacteria translocate across the blood–brain barrier and cause meningitis (Robinson et al. 2001). NFkB-induced expression of PAFr, and the observation that PAFr is elevated in the lungs of aged mice (see Fig. 5.3b) is further evidence that AAI in the elderly increases their susceptibility to infection.

5.4   Age-Related Defects in Immune Function

5.4.1   *Reduced Clinical Symptoms may be the Result of Impaired Toll-Like Receptor Function*

While chronic low-grade inflammation is associated with aging, a decline in immune function is also a hallmark of aging and leads to increased susceptibility to bacterial infections. One striking example of this phenomenon is the significant number of elderly with pneumonia who present without overt clinical symptoms. It is now known that aging is associated with a decline in TLR functions: age-related changes in TLR expression, TLR signaling, and TLR-dependent induction of proinflammatory cytokines has been shown by various investigators in both humans and mice and may explain why the innate and adaptive immune systems fail to become sufficiently activated. Renshaw et al. have shown decreased TLR expression on splenic and thio-glycollate-elicited macrophages from aged mice versus controls (Renshaw et al. 2002). Boehmer et al. have shown a reduction in the expression of mitogen-activated protein kinases such as JNK and their phosphorylation in macrophages isolated from the peritoneum of aged mice versus young controls (Boehmer et al. 2004). Finally, Duin et al. have demonstrated age-associated defects in the response of neutrophils isolated from the blood of aged human volunteers to an assortment of TLR ligands versus those isolated from healthy young adults (Van Duin et al. 2007). Thus, TLR dysfunction is one explanation for the lack of symptoms observed in some of the elderly with pneumonia. Future studies are warranted to determine if TLR defects occur in the lungs, their affect on alveolar macrophages, and to determine their impact during respiratory tract infection in an aged animal.

5.4.2   Other Age-Related Defects

Age-related immune dysfunctions are not limited to TLRs. For example, alveolar macrophages are decreased in number and are not efficient at presenting antigens to T-cells. Neutrophils have impaired chemotaxis and phagocytosis. Both macrophages and neutrophils demonstrate a decreased capacity to produce reactive oxygen species; nor is the adaptive immune system unaffected. Studies document a reduction in clonal expansion and function of antigen-specific T and B cells, a diminished ability to generate high-affinity protective antibodies against infectious agents, and a diminished and/or altered cytokine profile produced by T-helper cells. In summary, the elderly immune system becomes deficient at multiple levels and the collapse of these systems contributes to the susceptibility of the elderly to all infectious disease (Plackett et al. 2004).

5.5   Anti-inflammatory Drugs as Therapeutics

Worsening of clinical symptoms after initiation of antibiotic treatment during sepsis or meningitis has long been observed and has led to the use of corticosteroids and other agents concomitant or prior to the first antibiotic dose for immunosuppression. Cell wall active antibacterials (e.g., β-lactams) cause bacterial lysis and in the case of the pneumococcus, releases cell wall components and pneumolysin that enhance inflammation through TLR-2 and TLR-4. Bacteriostatic antibiotics, which inhibit RNA and protein synthesis, delay or even circumvent bacterial lysis, thus reducing inflammation. Given that much of the damage during pneumococcal infection is host-driven, investigators continue to examine the potential of anti-inflammatory drugs as therapeutics. While many, such as macrolides, have proven potential (Amsden 2005), we will discuss the use of statins as a possible prophylactic therapy.

5.5.1 Statins Inhibit NFkB Activation

Statins, 3-hydroxy-3-methylglutaryl coenzyme A (HMG-CoA) reductase inhibitors are among the most widely prescribed drugs in the United States. They are prescribed to treat hypercholesterolemia and inhibit the synthesis of cellular cholesterol. While statins can reduce plasma cholesterol by as much as by 30–55%, it is increasingly evident that statins also have potent anti-inflammatory properties that are independent of their lipid-lowering ability. Currently, it is believed that statins inhibit lipid raft formation and prenylation of signaling molecules, thereby inhibiting cell signal relaying and NFkB activation (Maron et al. 2000). Decreased NFkB activation during infection inhibits the production of inducible nitric oxide synthase (iNOS) and lowers the expression of acute-phase proteins, cytokines, and adhesion molecules. Statins also increase the production of endothelial nitric oxide synthase (eNOS). Unlike iNOS, which increases NO production at the nanomolar level and contributes to the development of shock, eNOS increases NO at a picomolar level and serves to preserve microvasculature tone and tight-junction integrity (McGown and Brookes 2007).

In the last 5 years more than 100 published findings have shown that statins inhibit NFkB activation in a wide variety of tissues and disease conditions. For example, Pravastatin inhibited endothelial cell activation after irradiation and decreased the resulting inflammatory response in mice (Gaugler et al. 2005). Similarly, Simvastatin inhibited NFkB activation and the expression of adhesion molecules in human endothelial cells activated with TNFα (Hilgendorff et al. 2003). Prospective and retrospective studies now indicate that statins are protective against acute bacterial infection. Statin therapy is associated with a decreased rate of sepsis (19% nonstatin group, 2.4% statin group, p = <0.001) (Almog et al. 2004), and increased survival in patients with multiple organ dysfunction syndrome (MODS) as a result of sepsis (mortality = 72% nonstatin group, 35% statin group, p = <0.001) (Schmidt et al. 2006). Finally, statin therapy has been associated with reduced mortality in patients with CAP (Mortensen et al. 2005) and associated with reduced risk of pneumonia in patients with diabetes (0.49 odds ratio/0.35–0.69, 95% confidence interval), a known risk group for IPD (Van de Garde et al. 2006). Thus, statin therapy offers potential prophylaxis for individuals who are at high risk for IPD, presumably by decreasing pIgR and PAFr expression. It currently remains unclear if statins may be used as a treatment during acute infection.

5.6 Summary

An abundance of evidence indicates that: (1) inflammation occurs in the elderly, (2) inflammation increases susceptibility to S. pneumoniae infection, (3) pneumococcal infection causes inflammation, and (4) excessive inflammation is detrimental. Thus, in the elderly, physiological factors are in place for the development of a positive feedback loop that contributes to patient mortality. Because inflammation underpins these mechanisms, therapies that block inflammation, such as statins, have the potential to protect against IPD.

References

Akira S, Sato S. Toll-like receptors and their signaling mechanisms. Scand J Infect Dis 2003;35:555–62.

Almog Y, Shefer A, Novack V, et al. Prior statin therapy is associated with a decreased rate of severe sepsis. Circulation 2004;110:880–5.

Amsden GW. Anti-inflammatory effects of macrolides – an underappreciated benefit in the treatment of community-acquired respiratory tract infections and chronic inflammatory pulmonary conditions? J Antimicrob Chemother 2005;55:10–21.

Antunes G, Evans SA, Lordan JL, et al. Systemic cytokine levels in community-acquired pneumonia and their association with disease severity. Eur Respir J 2002;20:990–5.

Armstrong L, Medford AR, Uppington KM, et al. Expression of functional toll-like receptor-2 and -4 on alveolar epithelial cells. Am J Respir Cell Mol Biol 2004;31:241–5.

Atkinson W, Hamborsky J, McIntyre L, et al. Pneumococcal disease. In: Centers for Disease Control and Prevention Epidemiology and Prevention of Vaccine-Preventable Diseases. Washington, DC: Public Health Foundation; 2007.

Becker S, Fenton MJ, Soukup JM. Involvement of microbial components and toll-like receptors 2 and 4 in cytokine responses to air pollution particles. Am J Respir Cell Mol Biol 2002;27:611–8.

Berry AM, Paton JC. Additive attenuation of virulence of Streptococcus pneumoniae by mutation of the genes encoding pneumolysin and other putative pneumococcal virulence proteins. Infect Immun 2000;68:133–40.

Berry AM, Paton JC, Hansman D. Effect of insertional inactivation of the genes encoding pneumolysin and autolysin on the virulence of Streptococcus pneumoniae type 3. Microb Pathog 1992;12:87–93.

Boehmer ED, Goral J, Faunce DE, et al. Age-dependent decrease in toll-like receptor 4-mediated proinflammatory cytokine production and mitogen-activated protein kinase expression. J Leukoc Biol 2004;75:342–9.

Braun JS, Sublett JE, Freyer D, et al. Pneumococcal pneumolysin and $H(2)O(2)$ mediate brain cell apoptosis during meningitis. J Clin Invest 2002;109:19–27.

Bruno ME, Kaetzel CS. Long-term exposure of the HT-29 human intestinal epithelial cell line to TNF causes sustained up-regulation of the polymeric Ig receptor and proinflammatory genes through transcriptional and posttranscriptional mechanisms. J Immunol 2005;174:7278–84.

Bruunsgaard H, Skinhoj P, Qvist J, et al. Elderly humans show prolonged in vivo inflammatory activity during pneumococcal infections. J Infect Dis 1999;180:551–4.

Bruunsgaard H, Pedersen M, Pedersen BK. Aging and proinflammatory cytokines. Curr Opin Hematol 2001;8:131–6.

Bruyn GA, van Furth R. Pneumococcal polysaccharide vaccines: indications, efficacy and recommendations. Eur J Clin Microbiol Infect Dis 1991;10:897–910.

Burns T, Abadi M, Pirofski LA. Modulation of the lung inflammatory response to serotype 8 pneumococcal infection by a human immunoglobulin m monoclonal antibody to serotype 8 capsular polysaccharide. Infect Immun 2005;73:4530–8.

Canvin JR, Marvin AP, Sivakumaran M, et al. The role of pneumolysin and autolysin in the pathology of pneumonia and septicemia in mice infected with a type 2 pneumococcus. J Infect Dis 1995;172:119–23.

Cundell DR, Tuomanen EI. Receptor specificity of adherence of Streptococcus pneumoniae to human type-II pneumocytes and vascular endothelial cells in vitro. Microb Pathog 1994;17:361–74.

Cundell DR, Gerard NP, Gerard C, et al. Streptococcus pneumoniae anchor to activated human cells by the receptor for platelet-activating factor. Nature 1995;377:435–8.

Dallaire F, Ouellet N, Bergeron Y, et al. Microbiological and inflammatory factors associated with the development of pneumococcal pneumonia. J Infect Dis 2001;184:292–300.

Dopazo J, Mendoza A, Herrero J, et al. Annotated draft genomic sequence from a Streptococcus pneumoniae type 19F clinical isolate. Microb Drug Resist 2001;7:99–125.

Dziarski R, Tapping RI, Tobias PS. Binding of bacterial peptidoglycan to CD14. J Biol Chem 1998;273:8680–90.

Dziarski R, Ulmer AJ, Gupta D. Interactions of CD14 with components of gram-positive bacteria. Chem Immunol 2000;74:83–107.

Edwards KM. Pneumococcal infections: therapeutic strategies and pitfalls. In: Tuomanen EI, Mitchell TJ, Morrison DA, Spratt BG, eds. The Pneumococcus. Washington, DC.: ASM; 2004:314–30.

Ershler WB. Interleukin-6: a cytokine for gerontologists. J Am Geriatr Soc 1993;41:176–81.

Fournier B, Philpott DJ. Recognition of Staphylococcus aureus by the innate immune system. Clin Microbiol Rev 2005;18:521–40.

French N, Nakiyingi J, Carpenter LM, et al. 23-valent pneumococcal polysaccharide vaccine in HIV-1-infected Ugandan adults: double-blind, randomised and placebo controlled trial. Lancet 2000;355:2106–11.

Gaugler MH, Vereycken-Holler V, Squiban C, et al. Pravastatin limits endothelial activation after irradiation and decreases the resulting inflammatory and thrombotic responses. Radiat Res 2005;163:479–87.

Glynn P, Coakley R, Kilgallen I, et al. Circulating interleukin 6 and interleukin 10 in community acquired pneumonia. Thorax 1999;54:51–5.

Granton JT, Grossman RF. Community-acquired pneumonia in the elderly patient. Clinical features, epidemiology, and treatment. Clin Chest Med 1993;14:537–53.

Gupta D, Kirkland TN, Viriyakosol S, et al. CD14 is a cell-activating receptor for bacterial peptidoglycan. J Biol Chem 1996;271:23310–6.

Gupta D, Wang Q, Vinson C, et al. Bacterial peptidoglycan induces CD14-dependent activation of transcription factors CREB/ATF and AP-1. J Biol Chem 1999;274:14012–20.

Gutierrez F, Masia M, Mirete C, et al. The influence of age and gender on the population-based incidence of community-acquired pneumonia caused by different microbial pathogens in a population-based prospective cohort study. J Infect 2006;53:166–74.

Hilgendorff A, Muth H, Parviz B, et al. Statins differ in their ability to block NF-kappaB activation in human blood monocytes. Int J Clin Pharmacol Ther 2003;41:397–401.

Hoskins J, Alborn WE, Jr., Arnold J, et al. Genome of the bacterium Streptococcus pneumoniae strain R6. J Bacteriol 2001;183:5709–17.

Houldsworth S, Andrew PW, Mitchell TJ. Pneumolysin stimulates production of tumor necrosis factor alpha and interleukin-1 beta by human mononuclear phagocytes. Infect Immun 1994;62:1501–3.

Janssens JP. Pneumonia in the elderly (geriatric) population. Curr Opin Pulm Med 2005;11:226–30.

Johnson JC, Jayadevappa R, Baccash PD, et al. Nonspecific presentation of pneumonia in hospitalized older people: age effect or dementia? J Am Geriatr Soc 2000;48:1316–20.

Kadioglu A, Gingles NA, Grattan K, et al. Host cellular immune response to pneumococcal lung infection in mice. Infect Immun 2000;68:492–501.

Kaetzel CS. Polymeric Ig receptor: defender of the fort or Trojan horse? Curr Biol 2001;11:R35–8.

Koivula I, Sten M, Makela PH. Risk factors for pneumonia in the elderly. Am J Med 1994;96:313–20.

Krabbe KS, Pedersen M, Bruunsgaard H. Inflammatory mediators in the elderly. Exp Gerontol 2004;39:687–99.

Lexau CA, Lynfield R, Danila R, et al. Changing epidemiology of invasive pneumococcal disease among older adults in the era of pediatric pneumococcal conjugate vaccine. JAMA 2005;294:2043–51.

Loeb M. Pneumonia in the elderly. Curr Opin Infect Dis 2004;17:127–30.

Luton F, Verges M, Vaerman JP, et al. The SRC family protein tyrosine kinase p62yes controls polymeric IgA transcytosis in vivo. Mol Cell 1999;4:627–32.

Malley R, Henneke P, Morse SC, et al. Recognition of pneumolysin by toll-like receptor 4 confers resistance to pneumococcal infection. Proc Natl Acad Sci USA 2003;100:1966–71.

Manukyan M, Triantafilou K, Triantafilou M, et al. Binding of lipopeptide to CD14 induces physical proximity of CD14, TLR2 and TLR1. Eur J Immunol 2005;35:911–21.

Marks M, Burns T, Abadi M, et al. Influence of neutropenia on the course of serotype 8 pneumococcal pneumonia in mice. Infect Immun 2007;75:1586–97.

Maron DJ, Fazio S, Linton MF. Current perspectives on statins. Circulation 2000;101:207–13.

McBean AM, Jung K, Hebert PL. Decreasing invasive pneumococcal disease in the elderly: a state-level analysis. Vaccine 2006;24:5609–14.

McGown CC, Brookes ZL. Beneficial effects of statins on the microcirculation during sepsis: the role of nitric oxide. Br J Anaesth 2007;98:163–75.

Meyer KC, Soergel P. Variation of bronchoalveolar lymphocyte phenotypes with age in the physiologically normal human lung. Thorax 1999;54:697–700.

Meyer KC, Ershler W, Rosenthal NS, et al. Immune dysregulation in the aging human lung. Am J Respir Crit Care Med 1996;153:1072–9.

Mortensen EM, Restrepo MI, Anzueto A, et al. The effect of prior statin use on 30-day mortality for patients hospitalized with community-acquired pneumonia. Respir Res 2005;6:82.

Mufson MA. Pneumococcal pneumonia. Curr Infect Dis Rep 1999;1:57–64.

Niederman MS, Mandell LA, Anzueto A, et al. Guidelines for the management of adults with community-acquired pneumonia. Diagnosis, assessment of severity, antimicrobial therapy, and prevention. Am J Respir Crit Care Med 2001;163:1730–54.

Orihuela CJ, Gao G, Francis KP, et al. Tissue-specific contributions of pneumococcal virulence factors to pathogenesis. J Infect Dis 2004;190:1661–9.

Paolisso G, Rizzo MR, Mazziotti G, et al. Advancing age and insulin resistance: role of plasma tumor necrosis factor-alpha. Am J Physiol 1998;275(2 Pt 1):E294–9.

Pichichero ME, Rennels MB, Edwards KM, et al. Combined tetanus, diphtheria, and 5-component pertussis vaccine for use in adolescents and adults. JAMA 2005;293:3003–11.

Plackett TP, Boehmer ED, Faunce DE, et al. Aging and innate immune cells. J Leukoc Biol 2004;76:291–9.

Pneumococcal vaccines. WHO position paper. Wkly Epidemiol Rec 1999;74:177–83.

Preventing pneumococcal disease among infants and young children. Recommendations of the Advisory Committee on Immunization Practices (ACIP). MMWR Recomm Rep 2000;49(RR-9):1–35.

Radin JN, Orihuela CJ, Murt G, et al. beta-Arrestin 1 participates in platelet-activating factor receptor-mediated endocytosis of Streptococcus pneumoniae. Infect Immun 2005; 73:6182–91.

Ratner AJ, Lysenko ES, Paul MN, et al. Synergistic proinflammatory responses induced by polymicrobial colonization of epithelial surfaces. Proc Natl Acad Sci USA 2005;102:3429–34.

Regev-Yochay G, Raz M, Dagan R, et al. Nasopharyngeal carriage of Streptococcus pneumoniae by adults and children in community and family settings. Clin Infect Dis 2004;38:632–9.

Renshaw M, Rockwell J, Engleman C, et al. Cutting edge: impaired toll-like receptor expression and function in aging. J Immunol 2002;169:4697–701.

Robinson KA, Baughman W, Rothrock G, et al. Epidemiology of invasive Streptococcus pneumoniae infections in the United States, 1995–1998: opportunities for prevention in the conjugate vaccine era. JAMA 2001;285:1729–35.

Rosenow C, Ryan P, Weiser JN, et al. Contribution of novel choline-binding proteins to adherence, colonization and immunogenicity of Streptococcus pneumoniae. Mol Microbiol 1997;25:819–29.

Saito T, Yamamoto T, Kazawa T, et al. Expression of toll-like receptor 2 and 4 in lipopolysaccharide-induced lung injury in mouse. Cell Tissue Res 2005;321:75–88.

Sarkar D, Fisher PB. Molecular mechanisms of aging-associated inflammation. Cancer Lett 2006;236:13–23.

Schmidt H, Hennen R, Keller A, et al. Association of statin therapy and increased survival in patients with multiple organ dysfunction syndrome. Intensive Care Med 2006;32:1248–51.

Seachrist JL, Ferguson SS. Regulation of G protein-coupled receptor endocytosis and trafficking by Rab GTPases. Life Sci 2003;74:225–35.

Shapiro ED, Berg AT, Austrian R, et al. The protective efficacy of polyvalent pneumococcal polysaccharide vaccine. N Engl J Med 1991;325:1453–60.

Silverman N, Maniatis T. NF-kappaB signaling pathways in mammalian and insect innate immunity. Genes Dev 2001;15:2321–42.

Sniadack DH, Schwartz B, Lipman H, et al. Potential interventions for the prevention of childhood pneumonia: geographic and temporal differences in serotype and serogroup distribution of sterile site pneumococcal isolates from children—implications for vaccine strategies. Pediatr Infect Dis J 1995;14:503–10.

Spencer NF, Poynter ME, Im SY, et al. Constitutive activation of NF-kappa B in an animal model of aging. Int Immunol 1997;9:1581–8.

Srivastava A, Henneke P, Visintin A, et al. The apoptotic response to pneumolysin is toll-like receptor 4 dependent and protects against pneumococcal disease. Infect Immun 2005;73:6479–87.

Takeda K, Kaisho T, Akira S. Toll-like receptors. Annu Rev Immunol 2003;21:335–76.

Tuomanen E. Attachment and invasion of the respiratory tract. In: Tuomanen E, Mitchell T, Morrison DA, Spratt BG, eds. The Pneumococcus. Washington, D.C.: ASM; 2004:221–37.

Tuomanen E, Rich R, Zak O. Induction of pulmonary inflammation by components of the pneumococcal cell surface. Am Rev Respir Dis 1987;135:869–74.

van de Garde EM, Hak E, Souverein PC, et al. Statin therapy and reduced risk of pneumonia in patients with diabetes. Thorax 2006;61:957–61.

van Duin D, Mohanty S, Thomas V, et al. Age-associated defect in human TLR-1/2 function. J Immunol 2007;178:970–5.

Weber JR, Freyer D, Alexander C, et al. Recognition of pneumococcal peptidoglycan: an expanded, pivotal role for LPS binding protein. Immunity 2003;19:269–79.

Whitney CG, Farley MM, Hadler J, et al. Decline in invasive pneumococcal disease after the introduction of protein-polysaccharide conjugate vaccine. N Engl J Med 2003;348:1737–46.

Xiao C, Ghosh S. NF-kappaB, an evolutionarily conserved mediator of immune and inflammatory responses. Adv Exp Med Biol 2005;560:41–5.

Yende S, Tuomanen EI, Wunderink R, et al. Preinfection systemic inflammatory markers and risk of hospitalization due to pneumonia. Am J Respir Crit Care Med 2005;172:1440–6.

Zhang JR, Mostov KE, Lamm ME, et al. The polymeric immunoglobulin receptor translocates pneumococci across human nasopharyngeal epithelial cells. Cell 2000;102:827–37.

Chapter 6
Nonspecific Removal of Sepsis Mediators

Xosé Luis Pérez-Fernandez, Joan Sabater Riera, and Rafael Mañez

6.1 Introduction

Sepsis is a growing clinical problem in our society, with an estimated annual incidence rate of above 300 cases per 100,000 people and mortality that exceeds 30% in those individuals suffering the disease (Esteban et al. 2007; Angus et al. 2001). Despite apparent recent successes in the treatment (Bernard et al. 2001), sepsis morbidity and mortality remain very high. This implies that new efforts are needed to translate to the clinical practice the huge information that preclinical research has generated in the past decade about the mechanisms of sepsis.

One of the problems is that sepsis entails multiple disorders in different organs and systems, the individual contribution of each one, or the dominance of a particular one, in the disease process being unclear. Initially, sepsis was considered a disorder due to an uncontrolled inflammatory response (Hotchkiss and Karl 2003). However, clinical interventions directed to the inflammatory elements did not reduce morbidity and mortality associated with the disease (Hotchkiss and Karl 2003). Since inflammation and coagulation are tightly linked, and sepsis-associated coagulopathy is almost universal in patients with severe sepsis, antithrombotic-targeted therapy has been clinically investigated with an apparent success, though controversial and limited (Costa et al. 2007; Nadel et al. 2007). Recent data also suggests that most deaths from sepsis are due to an extensive death of immune mediator cells (Hotchkiss and Nicholson 2006). Therefore, in 15 years we have moved from immunostimulation to immunosuppression as cause of sepsis, with one stop in coagulation disorders.

Are we talking about the same disease? Are all these findings different steps in the same disorder? Do they reflect a particular response of the host depending on genetic factors? Honestly, we do not know the answers to these questions yet. The numerous reasons proposed to explain the failure of the different therapies attempted in sepsis probably reflect more a hopeful expectation, such as targeting a single mediator would be enough to modify all events that take place in sepsis, than a real evidence. On the other hand, tailoring the therapy to an individual patient is something desired in medicine for many diseases, and sepsis is not an exception, but so far has been very difficult to achieve. In the meanwhile,

J. Rello, M.I. Restrepo (eds.) *Sepsis: New Strategies for Management.*
doi:10.1007/978-3-540-79001-3; © Springer-Verlag 2008

approaches addressed for nonspecific removal of sepsis mediators appear an attractive option to restore organism homeostasis and improve the morbidity and mortality of this disease.

6.2   Why a Nonspecific Approach?

The predominant theory for many years considered sepsis an uncontrolled production of inflammatory molecules as per the data generated in clinical and preclinal studies (Waage et al. 1987; Remick et al. 1987). This prompted several clinical trials with the goal of blocking tumor necrosis factor (TNF) or interleukin (IL-1) (Remick 2003). These trials did not show a significant improvement in patient survival, though a meta-analysis of TNF inhibitors suggested a better outcome in treated patients (Marshall 2003). An often explanation for the failure of these trials was that the anti-inflammatory agents were not administered quickly enough, but there may be others. An inflammatory mediator must be elevated and detectable to be implicated in the pathogenesis of sepsis. The problem is that cytokines and other inflammatory mediators may have considerable local effects without detectable changes at plasma levels (Remick 2007). Thus, a recent clinical trial in sepsis showed that neonates with sepsis improved after treatment with IL-1 receptor antagonist, even though IL-1 was not detected in plasma (Goldbach-Mansky et al. 2006), and recovery was associated with a decrease in IL-6 plasma levels.

Other studies have shown that intensive care unit (ICU) patients have reduced production of both TNF and IL-6 in response to endotoxin stimulation (Heagy et al. 2000, 2004), while IL-10 production was not impaired (Rigato and Salomao 2003). These data suggest that instead of a hyperinflammatory response, septic patients might present an anti-inflammatory or immunosuppressive response, which has been attributed to the apoptosis of cells of the innate and adaptive immune system (Hotchkiss and Nocholson 2006). Apoptosis causes the deletion of critical effector immune cells and the release of anti-inflammatory cytokines such as IL-10 and transforming growth factor-β (TGFβ), and suppresses the release of proinflammatory cytokines. However, similarly to what happened with anti-inflammatory treatments, use of immunostimulants such as granulocyte macrophage colony-stimulating factor or interferon-γ did not modify survival in septic patients (Root et al. 2003; Dries et al. 1994).

Something analogous to what happens with inflammation occurs with the dysfunction of coagulation in sepsis. Activation of the coagulation cascade can be produced by several noninfectious insults, such as thermal injury, pancreatitis, and trauma. In this case, the activation of coagulation is associated with an inflammatory response through TNF-α release and complement activation (Esmon 2000). In sepsis, along with the activation of coagulation through the proinflammatory cascade, there is also a direct activation of coagulation by infectious toxins that upregulate tissue factor (TF) in endothelial cells, leading to the formation of thrombin and fibrin clots (Tapper and Herwald 2000). However, the procoagulant activity in sepsis is not limited only to the endothelium, since TF is also present in circulating activated monocytes. Thrombin is also generated by these cells, allowing an unlimited supply of TF and a generalized activation of coagulation. This leads to the depletion of natural antithrombotic factors, such as protein C, antithrombin (AT), and TF pathway inhibitor (TFPI), turning the hemostatic system into an appropriate target for sepsis intervention. Unfortunately, as what happened with the anti- and proinflammatory treatments, clinical studies failed to demonstrate a benefit for recombinant TFPI or AT (Warren et al. 2001), and only activated protein C appears to yield a limited benefit.

All these data suggest that the inflammatory and coagulation responses in sepsis are multifaceted, not clearly classified as augmented or decreased, and probably with more unknown elements than those that we know. This has led to the rationale for nonspecific elimination of circulating mediators in sepsis by continuous extracorporeal removal mechanisms. The consideration of these techniques as potential therapeutic options in septic patients is also a consequence of the advances of technology. Continuous renal replacement therapies (CRRTs) have progressively evolved from a therapy of last resort for acute renal failure to a standardized technique for critically ill patients. This has created a new scenario where the CRRT is foreseen as a possible therapeutic approach in critical care patients with multiple organ dysfunction syndrome (MODS), regardless of whether the patients exhibit a renal failure or not (Ricc et al. 2004).

6.3 Continuous Renal Replacement Therapy

Replacement of the renal function may be performed through hemodialysis (HD) or hemofiltration (HF). HD is achieved by diffusive clearance along with a concentration gradient from blood to a dialysate through a semipermeable membrane. Small molecules (urea, creatinine, potassium) diffuse rapidly and are efficiently removed, whereas larger solutes that diffuse poorly are cleared slowly. HD is performed intermittently for the treatment of patients with chronic renal failure (CRF) or acute renal failure (ARF) without hemodynamic compromise to restore metabolic and/or fluid balance.

HF is based on convective mass transport. A transmembrane pressure drives both fluid and solutes through a membrane selected for its high hydraulic permeability, allowing removal of larger solutes than HD. Convective removal of a solute (sieving coefficient) depends on transmembrane pressure (TMP), on molecular weight (MW) and structure of the solute, as well as on the cutoff point of the membrane. HF may be performed intermittently but it is usually executed as CRRT, namely continuous veno-venous hemofiltration (CVVH). CRRT includes other techniques also, such as the continuous veno-venous hemodialysis (CVVHD), which uses diffusion as the main mechanism to remove solutes, and continuous veno-venous hemodiafiltration (CVVHDF), which combines both HD and HF. Most of the filters used in these techniques have an adsorption property, which is defined as the molecular adherence to the surface or interior of a semipermeable membrane. Thus, CRRT may include three types of depurative mechanisms: convection, diffusion, and adsorption.

Different strategies have been investigated for renal replacement in critical care patients, making CRRT the most extensively used therapy in clinical practice. The reason is that many patients in ICU are hemodynamically unstable and cannot tolerate the subtraction of the blood volume required for intermittent HD. Despite that some authors settled that alternate-day HD should no longer be considered adequate for critically ill patients with acute renal failure (Schiffl et al. 2002), no study has obtained conclusive results of the benefits of CRRT versus intermitent HD (Kellum and Bellomo 2000; Vinsonneau et al. 2006; Ronco and Bellomo 2007).

A high percentage of septic patients develop ARF, exceeding 50% in the case of septic shock. Combination of sepsis and ARF usually leads to MODS, which is associated with more than 80% mortality. Thus, many septic patients require an intensive care support that most of the times includes mechanical ventilation and renal replacement therapy (Schrier and Wang 2004). CVVHD or CVVHDF have been proposed for renal replacement in septic patients, based on a better control of azotemia (Ricci et al. 2006; Saudan et al. 2006; Page et al. 2005). Other authors recommended the use of slow extended dialysis, which appears to be associated with equivalent cardiovascular stability and solute control as CRRT in septic patients (Kumar et al. 2004). However, CRRT have become extensively used in septic patients with renal failure because of their apparent ability to remove, along with the small MW solutes, middle MW molecules that would include cytokines and other sepsis mediators (Kellum et al. 1998).

6.4 CRRT and Cytokine Removal

Nonspecific elimination of circulating cytokines and other inflammatory mediators by CRRT has been a matter of controversy ever since it was first proposed. In 1976, Burton created the term *hemofiltration*, and one year later Kramer developed the continuous arteriovenous hemofiltration (CAVH) technique (Kramer et al. 1977), which used a systemic arteriovenous pressure difference in an extracorporeal circuit to continuously produce an ultrafiltrate. The limited capacity of this procedure to remove nephrotoxins led to the development of pump-driven techniques (Peachey et al. 1998; Storck et al. 1991). In 1991, CAVH was compared to pump-driven hemofiltration (PDHF), showing a better survival rate in the PDHF group that appeared related to a faster elimination of toxic mediators (Storck et al. 1991). These would include nephrotoxins and other toxins as suggested by the improvement in cardiovascular function with HF observed in animals after endotoxin injection and the impairment of hemodynamics in healthy animals with the infusion of the *septic ultrafiltrate* (Grootendorst et al. 1992).

Complications related to the arterial access lead to the development of veno-venous pump-driven techniques which have become extensively used for CRRT in intensive care units (Bellomo et al. 1993a,b). The expansion of these techniques was associated with the introduction of biocompatible membranes in the procedures that decreased the generation of inflammatory mediators by the system itself (Schiffl et al. 1994). In this setting, Bellomo et al. suggested that CRRT might remove cytokines (TNF-α and IL-1) from the circulation of septic patients (Bellomo et al. 1993b).

Since then, several studies have shown the presence of inflammatory mediators in the ultrafiltrate fluid from septic patients with CRRT. However, a few demonstrated a significant decrease in plasma concentrations of these mediators with the ultrafiltrate usually removed for renal replacement (Table 6.1) (Heering et al. 1997; Sander et al. 1997; Hoffmann et al. 1995). This discrepancy between the presence of inflammatory mediators in ultrafiltrate fluid and their lack of reduction in plasma suggest a constant production of mediators during sepsis. Similarly, HF has been associated with hemodynamic improvements in critically ill patients and animal models of acute endotoxic shock without a correlation with the decrease in cytokine plasma concentrations (Sanchez-Izquierdo et al. 1997; Kamijo et al. 2000; Rogiers et al. 1999; Mink et al. 1999).

Table 6.1 Mediators clearance with CRRT

Author	Study	Modality	Membrane	Ultrafiltrate dose	Ultrafiltrate analysis	Plasma reduction
Rogiers et al. (1999)	Dogs	HVHF	PS	6 l/h	TNF	No
Bellomo (2000)	Dogs	HVHF	AN69	80 ml/kg/h	ET-1, PGF1α	No
Bellomo (1993b)	Humans	CVVHD	AN69	–	TNF IL-1	No
Sanchez-Izquierdo Riera (1997)	Humans	CVVH	AN69	300 ml/h	TNF, IL-6	No
Hoffmann. et al (1995)	Humans	CVVH	PA	2 l/h	TNF, IL-2, IL-6	C3a
Journois et al. (1996)	Humans (pediatric)	HVHF	AN69	5 l/m²	TNF, IL-10	IL-1, IL-6, IL-8
Heering et al. (1997)	Humans	CVVH	PS	1 l/h	TNF, IL-1, IL-2R, IL-8	No
Sander et al. (1997)	Humans	CVVH	AN69	1 l/h	TNF, IL-6	No
De Vriese et al. (1999)	Humans	CVVH	AN69	1.5–2.7 l/h	TN IL-6, IL-1	No
Kamijo et al. (2000)	Humans	CVVH	AN69	500–1,000 ml/h	IL-6	No
Cole et al. (2001)	Humans	HVHF	AN69	80 ml/kg/h	C3, C5, IL-10	Transitory changes
Ghani et al. (2006)	Humans	HVHF	PS	100 ml/kg/h	IL-6	IL-6

AN69 polyacrylonitrile; *HVHF* high volume hemofiltration; *PA* polyamide; *PS* polysulphone; *ET* endothelin; *PG* prostaglandin

Convective techniques of CRRT (CVVH) have been considered more efficacious for cytokine removal than diffusive techniques (CVVHD) in septic patients (Table 6.1) (Kellum et al. 1998). The rationale is that HF might remove higher MW molecules than HD. This benefit of convective techniques has been recently argued by one study that suggested no benefit from CVVH compared to CVVHD for the removal of both small and middle MW molecules, which include cytokines (Ricci et al. 2006). However, it should be noted that the clearance of middle MW molecules was higher with CVVH than with CVVHD, though it did not reach the statistical significance ($p = 0.055$). On the other hand, the effect of CRRT on cytokine removal and blood pressure appeared not only be explained by convective or diffusive clearance of the mediators, suggesting other mechanisms of clearance (Bellomo et al. 2000). This led to propose adsorption to the membrane as the main clearance mechanism of cytokines, being most pronounced immediately after installation of a new membrane and decreasing steadily thereafter by a rapid saturation of the membrane (Goldfarb and Golper 1994; De Vriese et al. 1999). Nevertheless, in this case, the same study that questioned the benefit of the convective versus diffusive techniques has presented more solid data that minimizes the contribution of adsorption to remove inflammatory mediators (Ricci et al. 2006).

Therefore, mediators related to sepsis may be found in the ultrafiltrate fluid from septic patients during CRRT, suggesting their removal by this technique, though the plasma level of these mediators does not change. Then, why do hemodynamics and clinics improve with CRRT in septic patients? Ronco et al. proposed the "peak concentration hypothesis" to explain these events. This considers the response to sepsis in a network perspective, where absolute values are less relevant than relative ones and small decreases might induce major balance changes. Thus, the clinical and hemodynamic benefits of CRRT in sepsis may be due to the ability of this technique to lower peaks of mediators such as the pro- and anti-inflammatory, pro- and anticoagulant, and likely others, reducing their toxic effects and leading to a nearly normal inmunohomeostasis (Ronco et al. 2001).

6.5   CRRT in Sepsis

Several factors influence the potential beneficial effects of CRRT in sepsis. These include the amount of ultrafiltrate, the moment of initiation, and the permeability of the filter used for CRRT.

6.6   Ultrafiltrate Dose

In chronic hemodialysis patients, hemodialysis dose might affect morbidity and mortality (Gotch and Sargent 1985). A similar correlation between outcome (survival) and dose of treatment with CRRT (volume of ultrafiltrate) was also suggested in ischemic or septic ARF (Storck et al. 1991). Subsequently, animal studies confirmed this link between dose of ultrafiltrate and survival in sepsis (Table 6.2) (Rogiers et al. 1999; Yekebas et al. 2001).

Table 6.2 Clinical response to CRRT

Author	Study	Modality	Ultrafiltrate dose	Clinical improvement
Grootendorst et al. (1992)	Pigs	HVHF	150 ml/kg/h	HMD, RESP
Lee et al. (1998)	Pigs	HVHF	50–75 ml/kg/h	RESP, SURV
Rogiers et al. (1999)	Dogs	HVHF	200 ml/kg/h	HMD
Bellomo (2000)	Dogs	HVHF	80 ml/kg/h	HMD
Yekebas (2001)	Pigs	HVHF	100 ml/kg/h	HMD, SURV
Hoffmann et al. (1995)	Humans	CVVH	2 l/h	HMD
Journois et al. (1996)	Humans (pediatric)	HVHF	5 l/m²	RESP
Sander et al. (1997)	Humans	CVVH	1 l/h	No improvement
Heering et al. (1997)	Humans	CVVH	1 l/h	HMD
Oudemans-van Straaten et al. (1999)	Humans	HVHF	3.8 l/h	HMD, SURV
Kamijo et al. (2000)	Humans	HVVC	500–1,000 ml/h	HMD
Ronco (2000)	Humans	HVHF	45 ml/kg/h	SURV
Honore et al. (2000)	Humans	HVHF	116 ml/Kg/h	HMD, SURV
Cole et al. (2001)	Humans	HVHF	80 ml/kg/h	HMD
Cornejo et al. (2006)	Humans	HVHF	100 ml/kg/h	HMD, SURV
Ratanarat et al. (2005)	Humans	PHVHF	85 ml/kg/h (6–8 h) + 35 ml/kg/h (16–18 h)	HMD, SURV
Ghani et al. (2006)	Humans	PHVHF	100 ml/kg/h (6 h) + 35 ml/kg/h (18 h)	HMD

HMD hemodynamic; *RESP* respiratory; *SURV* survival; *PHVHF* pulse HVHF

The largest clinical trial evaluating the impact of different ultrafiltration doses in critically ill patients with ARF, either septic or not, randomized patients to ultrafiltration rates of 20 ml/kg/h (group 1), 35 ml/kg/h (group 2), and 45 ml/kg/h (group 3). The survival rate was significantly lower in group 1 (41%) compared to groups 2 (57%) and 3 (58%), indicating that a minimal renal dose of 35 ml/kg/h is required to replace renal function in critically ill patients with ARF. In the subgroup of patients with sepsis, survival was 47% in group 3 compared to 18% in group 2 and 25% in group 1. Though the differences did not reach statistical significance, the authors postulated that sepsis patients might benefit from an ultrafiltrate dose >35 ml/kg/h (sepsis dose) (Ronco et al. 2000). Since then, different doses of hemofiltration have been investigated in patients with septic shock (Table 6.2).

In a group of septic shock patients with organ dysfunction, the hemodynamic parameters increased regularly during HF treatment with ultrafiltration rates between 40 and 60 ml/kg/h. The improvement of hemodynamics was associated with a beneficial effect on 28-day mortality (46% vs. 70%) (Joannes-Boyau et al. 2004). In addition, the efficacy of HF with ultrafiltration of 35 l in 4 h was evaluated in patients with refractory septic shock. Improvement in hemodynamics was observed in 11 of the 20 patients studied. Of these, 9 (81%) were alive on day 28, while all nonresponders died within one day. The observed mortality was significantly lower than the APACHE II, SAPS II predicted mortality, being patient's weight and the time from ICU admission to HF the factors associated with a clinical response. The fact that the weight was a factor associated with improvement emphasizes the relevance of the volume of ultrafiltration, since the study used a fixed ultrafiltration rate per hour instead of adjusting this to patient's weight (Honore et al. 2000). Other studies investigated different doses of ultrafiltration (85, 80, or 70 ml/kg/h during 6–12 h) (Oudemans-van Straaten et al. 1999; Cole et al. 2001; Ratanarat et al. 2005; Cornejo et al. 2006; Jiang et al. 2005), suggesting an improvement in hemodynamics and short-term patient survival compared to the conventional doses used in CRRT for ARF (Table 6.2). Bouman has summarized the different doses of ultrafiltration in three groups (Bouman et al. 2007):

– Low volume hemofiltration (LVHF): <30 ml/kg/h
– High volume hemofiltration (HVHF): 30–50 ml/kg/h
– Very high volume hemofiltration (VHVHF): >50 ml/kg/h

It should be noted that the concentration of mediators in the ultrafiltrate in studies with HVHF and VHVHF has shown inconsistent results (Table 6.1). Thus, some studies found an increase for removal of several cytokines, along with a drop in their plasma levels, in HVHF or VHVHF compared to LVHF for CRRT (Journois et al. 1996; Ghani et al. 2006). This fall in cytokines was not always associated with better hemodynamic effects in HVHF or VHVHF compared to LVHF (De Vriese et al. 1999). In contrast, other studies found a level of cytokines in the ultrafiltrate of HVHF negligible, and suggested adsorption as the major mechanism for mediator removal with these techniques (Cole et al. 2001). These variations may reflect particular differences with the HF methods or the technical difficulties involving the analysis of cytokines.

HVUF or VHVUF are not innocuous to the patients and may be associated with problems related to the vascular access and others such as hypothermia or ionic disorders. In addition, it requires a rapid change in drug dosing to compensate all the drugs that will undergo an extracorporeal clearance. On the other hand, when the filtration fraction (FF: the ratio between ultrafiltration and plasma flow) exceeds 30% with these techniques, TMP gradient progressively increased and membrane fouling occurred. This complication might be avoided by using the replacement solution before passage through the filter (predilution), though it might reduce efficiency compared with dilution after passage through the filter at similar ultrafiltration volumes. Finally, HVUF and VHVUF are expensive techniques that need a very well-trained team to perform. In this setting, short intermittent VHVUF sessions and maintenance with a HVUF rate around 35 ml/kg/h appear as the best way to balance the potential benefits and adverse effects of these techniques in septic patients with ARF. The problem is that the best dose and period for VHVHF have not been defined yet.

6.7   When CRRT Should Begin?

Sepsis is a "continuum" process that may develop MODS. Early antibiotics and hemodynamic goal-directed therapy (EGDT) are included in actual practice guidelines because they have proven a benefit for septic patients (Dellinger et al. 2004).

It seems reasonable to consider that removing or reducing the peak of mediators in an early phase of the sepsis may avoid MODS instauration. Experimental animal studies have confirmed this postulate showing that early HF treatment increases survival (Mink et al. 1999). The problem is that in experimental studies HF techniques are started before or shortly after the microbial challenge, whereas in clinical practice CRRT is started when shock and ARF are already established. The exception may be one study in patients with pancreatitis where HF was performed without ARF. It showed that HVUF and early treatment (within 48 h after onset of abdominal pain) was associated with significantly better survival that in the group of patients with late (96 h) LVUF (Jiang et al. 2005).

Several parameters have been studied for an earlier indication of CRRT in critically ill patients. These include the initiation of CRRT with a BUN < 60 mg/dl, which improved the survival of trauma patients with ARF compared to beginning with a greater renal dysfunction. As we indicated previously, the time from ICU admission to HVUF was significantly shorter in septic patients with refractory shock that improved with the treatment (<7 h) than in nonresponders (>12 h) (Gettings et al. 1999; Piccinni et al. 2006). Interestingly, two responders with delayed times (>12 h) died despite an improvement in the hemodynamic status, suggesting that even though cardiovascular reserve may be present, delay in treatment may lead to the development of a lethal injury (Honore et al. 2000). Other authors have used the acute respiratory failure commonly present in septic patients to initiate HF. When PaO_2/FiO_2 ratio was lower than 250, CVVH improved survival compared to an historical control group (Weksler et al. 2001). The exception to these studies is the one from Boumann that did not find differences in survival nor in recovery of renal function in severely ill patients with ARF with early (7 h) HVUF versus late (42 h) LVUF (Bouman et al. 2002).

In summary, early CRRT is associated with hemodynamic improvement and an apparent better survival rate in septic patients developing ARF. The problem is that for the moment there is no agreement about what indicator should be used for the initiation of therapy. On the other hand, there is a lack of studies analyzing HF in patients without ARF, since the majority of studies analyze early therapy HF in patients with at least established acute renal injury, which already implies the presence of MODS. The preliminary results obtained in the few studies that attempted HF without renal dysfunction warrant the application of these techniques to septic and other critically ill patients, if they can prove a benefit in prospective randomized clinical trials.

6.8 Membrane and Pore Size

Both membrane and solute characteristics (geometry, charge, MW, and protein binding) determine the degree of removal by ultrafiltration and adsorption in HF and HD. Important membrane-related determinants are pore characteristics (size, distribution, and density), pH, charge, and surface (Clark et al. 1999).

For some membranes, in particular the negatively charged polyacrylonitrile (AN69) membrane, adsorption appeared to be the main mechanism of mediator removal (De Vriese et al. 1999; Kellum and Bellomo 2000), though a recent study has questioned this effect (Ricci et al. 2006).

Filter permeability may dramatically influence the removal of plasma mediators. Conventional membranes usually have a pore size of about 5 nm, allowing the removal of molecules up to a MW of about 30 kDa. High cutoff membranes have pore sizes of about 10 nm, allowing the elimination of molecules with MW up to 50 kDa. The use of high cutoff membranes to increase cytokine removal has been discussed since it was first proposed. An animal septic model compared 100 kDa with 50-kDa pore size filters for HF, showing an increased survival rate in the 100-kDa group (8 times higher), though it was associated with an increased protein concentration in the ultrafiltrate (Lee et al. 1998).

The impact of filter permeability in the treatment of septic patients is unclear. In vitro studies using large filter pore size (100 kDa) for HF showed a significantly better clearance of cytokines by an augment of ultrafiltration rate from 1 to 6 l/h, without changes in the albumin clearance (Uchino et al. 2002). In a small observational study, intermittent HF with high cutoff membranes (HCOM–HF; in vitro cutoff of 100 kDa) led to a slight improvement of organ failure in 16 patients with septic shock and ARF combined with high IL-6 removal. However, there was a cumulative protein loss of almost 7.6 g/12 h (Morgera et al. 2003). The same authors performed a small randomized controlled trial in 30 patients with sepsis comparing HF with standard membranes (30 kDa) with HCOM–HF (60 kDa). Ultrafiltrate dose was 2.5 l/h in both groups. HCOM–HF was superior to HF allowing bigger decrease in norepinephrine dose and higher cytokine removal (IL-1 and IL-6) with significant decline of cytokine plasma levels (Morgera et al. 2006). Other study compared HD with HCOM membranes (HCOM–HD) during 4 h and HD with high flux during 4 h, in septic patients with ARF. HCOM–HD, but not HD with high flux, achieved substantial diffusive clearance of several cytokines (IL-6, IL-8, and IL-10). However, during HCOM–HD, cumulative albumin loss into the effluent was 7.7 g versus less than 1.0 g for HD with high flux (Haase et al. 2007). All these data suggest that HCOM could be a good option to increase cytokine removal. The main drawback of this method is the loss of proteins and its associated complications. Whether the benefit of HCOM may be added to that achieved with other strategies such as HVUF rates is unclear for the moment.

6.9 Other Therapies

In an attempt to increase cytokine removal, new strategies have been proposed: Total plasma exchange tries to replace *bad molecules by good molecules* with plasma transfusion; adsorption therapies with special cartridges aim to increase cytokine removal; and nonselective extracorporeal therapies like coupled plasma filtration adsorption (CPFA) combine both adsorption and convection techniques.

6.10   Plasmapheresis

Plasma exchange therapies (PE) separate plasma from whole blood by centrifugation or filtration mechanisms, and replace with human plasma. Plasma replacement could be a good option in septic patients because of the potential benefits of factor replacement. Experience in septic patients with PE is reduced, though most of the studies showed beneficial effects. Stegmayr et al. used PE as rescue therapy in 76 patients with severe MOF observing an increase in survival (86% vs. 33% APACHE II expected survival) (Stegmayr et al. 2003). The largest published trial included 106 septic patients and was associated with a decreased mortality in PE group of 20% (33% vs. 53.8%) (Busund et al. 2002). Finally, in pediatric patients with proved infection, PE was associated with a trend toward fewer organs failing, though it did not have an impact on mortality (Reeves et al. 1999).

6.11   Adsorption Techniques

These methods use cartridges containing materials such as resin-coated beads or fibers that bind the desired mediators. Endotoxin is one of the most important mediators of sepsis that have been targeted for adsorption. Multiple methods of removing endotoxin from blood or plasma have been developed utilizing various ligands such as polymyxin B, albumin, ofloxacin, bactericidal/permeability-increasing protein, endotoxin inhibitor, and cationic antibacterial protein 18 (Nillson et al. 2005).

Major clinical experience is related to the use of polymixin B cartridges (PMX-F) in gram negative infections. A recent meta-analysis including over 1,425 septic patients (978 treated with PMX-F) observed improvement in hemodynamics, PaO_2/FiO_2 ratio, endotoxin removal, and mortality in patients treated with the cartridges However, possible publication bias and lack of binding lead to the conclusion that further studies are needed to confirm the potential benefits of this therapy (Cruz et al. 2007).

6.12   Coupled Plasma Filtration Adsorption

Coupled plasma filtration adsorption (CPFA) is a blood purification technique in which blood passes through a plasmafilter separating a predetermined percentage of plasma. This plasma continues through a cartridge that removes mediators via nonselective adsorption. Plasma is then returned to combine with blood that subsequently can pass through a hemofilter for CRRT if needed. This technique showed in animal models a reduction in cytokine plasma concentrations and improvement in survival (Tetta et al. 2000). Clinical studies reported hemodynamic and gas exchange improvements with CPFA treatment (Formica et al. 2003). The main limitation of this technique is the lack of comparative studies with HF or HD, which does not allow us to conclude whether CPFA may give an additional benefit to the latter techniques or not.

Our own group, in a small uncontrolled trial, treated ten septic shock patients with severe MOF with either CPFA or HF with HVUF, observing a similar hemodynamic and gas exchange response in both groups (Perez et al. 2007).

6.13 Conclusion

Sepsis is the major cause of mortality in critically ill patients. The physiopathology pathways of the disease are complex and incompletely understood even now. Adequate and early antibiotic administration, infection focus eradication, and EGDT, continue to be the main cornerstones of sepsis therapy. Interventions designed to block the synthesis or the action of a particular component of the sepsis cascades have been attempted in the last years, but have not achieved the expected benefits.

CRRT in septic patients who develop ARF have produced benefits that go beyond the replacement of renal function. Peak reduction of cytokines and other sepsis mediators have been proposed to be responsible for the improvements observed in septic patients with CRRT. Ultrafiltrate dose, filter pore size, and membrane adsorption properties appear to be the issues that may convert CRRT in a therapeutic alternative to septic patients. Thus, ultrafiltration of at least 35 ml/kg/h should be the regular practice in critically ill patients when CRRT is needed, regardless of whether the patients are septic or not. The use of higher doses of ultrafiltration and high cutoff filters require more investigation and standardization before they can be recommended. For the moment, CRRT with short intermittent VHUF sessions (6–8 h) and maintenance with a HVUF rate around 35 ml/kg/h appear the best way to balance the potential benefits and adverse effects of these techniques in septic patients with renal injury or ARF.

Scientific evidence is too low to recommend the use of continuous replacement therapies as adjunctive treatment for septic patients without ARF. Similarly, the use of plasma exchange and adsorption techniques is a promising field but need to be compared to CRRT to appreciate the potential benefits. However, the potential benefit of the continuous replacement therapies and other blood exchange techniques to treat septic and other critically ill patients regardless of renal failure constitutes one of the more appealing therapeutic approaches for the critical care medicine in the twenty-first century.

References

Angus DC, Linde-Zwirble WT, Lidicker J, et al. Epidemiology of severe sepsis in the United States: analysis of incidence, outcome, and associated costs of care. Crit Care Med 2001; 29:1303–10.

Bellomo R, Tipping P, Boyce N. Prospective comparative study of continuous arteriovenous hemodiafiltration and continuous venovenous emodiafiltration in critically ill patients. Am J Kidney Dis 1993a; 21:400–4.

Bellomo R, Tipping P, Boyce N. Continuous veno-venous hemofiltration with dialysis removes cytokines from the circulation of septic patients. Crit Care Med 1993b; 21:522–6.

Bellomo R, Kellum JA, Gandhi CR, et al. The effect of intensive plasma water exchange by hemofiltration on hemodynamics and soluble mediators in canine endotoxemia. Am J Respir Crit Care Med 2000; 161:1429–36.

Bernard GR, Vincent JL, Laterre PF, et al. Evaluation in severe sepsis (PROWESS) study group: efficacy and safety of recombinant human activated protein C for severe sepsis. N Engl J Med 2001; 344:699–709.

Bouman CSC, Oudemans-van Straaten HM, Tijssen JPG, et al. Effects of early high-volume continuous venovenous hemofiltrationon survival and recovery of renal function in intensive care patients with acute renal failure: a prospective, randomized trial. Crit Care Med 2002; 30:2205–11.

Bouman CSC, Oudemans-van Straaten HM, Schultz MJ, et al. Hemofiltration in sepsis and systemic inflammatory response syndrome: the role of dosing and timing. J Crit Care 2007; 22:1–12.

Busund R, Koukline V, Utrobin U, et al. Plasmapheresis in severe sepsis and septic shock: a prospective, randomized, controlled trial. Intensive Care Med 2002; 28:1434–9.

Clark WR, Hamburger RJ, Lysaght MJ. Effect of membrane composition and structure on solute removal and biocompatibility in hemodialysis. Kidney Int 1999; 56:2005–15.

Cole L, Bellomo R, Journois D, et al. High-volume haemofiltration in human septic shock. Intensive Care Med 2001; 27:978–86.

Cornejo R, Downey P, Castro R, et al. High-volume hemofiltration as salvage therapy in severe hyperdynamic septic shock. Intensive Care Med 2006; 32:713–22.

Costa V, Brophy JM. Drotrecogin alfa (activated) in severe sepsis: a systematic review and new cost-effectiveness analysis. BMC Anesthesiol 2007; 7:5.

Cruz DN, Perazella MA, Bellomo R, et al. Effectiveness of polymyxin B-immobilized fiber column in sepsis: a systematic review. Crit Care 2007; 20:R47.

Dellinger RP, Carlet JM, Masur H, et al. Surviving sepsis campaign: guidelines for management of severe sepsis and septic shock. Intensive Care Med 2004; 30:536–55.

De Vriese AS, Colardyn FA, Philipp JJ, et al. Cytokine removal during continuous hemofiltration in septic patients. J Am Soc Nephrol 1999; 10:846–53.

Dries DJ, Jurkovich GJ, Maier RV, et al. Effect of interferon gamma on infection-related death in patients with severe injuries. A randomized, doubled-blind, placebo-controlled trial. Arch Surg 1994; 129:1031–41.

Esmon CT. Does inflammation contribute to thrombotic events? Haemostasis 2000; 30(Suppl 2): 34–40.

Esteban A, Frutos-Vivar F, Ferguson ND, et al. Sepsis incidence and outcome: contrasting the intensive care unit with the hospital ward. Crit Care Med 2007; 35:1284–9.

Formica M, Olivieri C, Livigni S, et al. Hemodynamic response to coupled plasmafiltration-adsorption in human septic shock. Intensive Care Med 2003; 29:703–8.

Gettings LG, Reynolds HN, Scalea T. Outcome in post-tramatic acute renal failure when continuous renal replacement therapy is applied early vs late. Intensive Care Med 1999; 25:805–13.

Ghani RA, Zainudin S, Ctokong N, Rahman AF, et al. Serum IL-6 and IL-1-ra with sequential organ failure assessment scores in septic patients receiving high-volume haemofiltration and continuous venovenous haemofiltration. Nephrology 2006; 11:386–93.

Goldbach-Mansky R, Dailey NJ, Canna SW, et al. Neonatal-onset multisystem inflammatory disease responsive to interleukin-1 beta inhibition. N Engl J Med 2006; 355:581–92.

Goldfarb S, Golper TA. Proinflammatory cytokines and hemofiltration membranes. J Am Soc Nephrol 1994; 5:228–32.

Gotch FA, Sargent JA. A mechanistic analysis of the National Cooperative Dialysis Study (NCDS). Kidney Int 1985; 28:526–34.

Grootendorst AF, van Bommel EF, van der Hoven B, et al. High volume hemofiltration improves right ventricular function in endotoxin-induced shock in the pig. Intensive Care Med 1992; 18:235–40.

Haase M, Bellomo R, Baldwin I. Hemodialysis membrane with a high-molecular-weight cutoff and cytokine levels in sepsis complicated by acute renal failure: a phase 1 randomized trial. Am J Kidney Dis 2007; 50:296–304.

Heagy W, Hansen C, Nieman K. Impaired ex vivo lipopolysaccharide-stimulated whole blood tumor necrosis factor production may identify "septic" intensive care unit patients. Shock 2000; 14:271–6.

Heagy W, Nieman K, Hansen C, et al. Lower levels of whole blood LPS-stimulated cytokine release are associated with poorer clinical outcomes in surgical ICU patients. Surg Infect 2004; 4:171–80.

Heering P, Morgera S, Schmitz FJ, et al. Cytokine removal and cardiovascular hemodynamics in septic patients with continuous venovenous hemofiltration. Intensive Care Med 1997; 23:288–96.

Hoffmann JN, Hartl WH, Deppisch R, et al. Hemofiltration in human sepsis: evidence for the elimination of immunomodulatory substances. Kidney Int 1995; 48:1563–70.

Honore PM, Jamez J, Wauthier M, et al. Prospective evaluation of short-term, high-volume isovolemic hemofiltration on the hemodynamic course and outcome in patients with intractable circulatory failure resulting from septic shock. Crit Care Med 2000; 28:3581–7.

Hotchkiss RS, Karl IE. The pathophysiology and treatment of sepsis. N Engl J Med 2003; 348:138–50.

Hotchkiss RS, Nicholson DW. Apoptosis and caspases regulate death and inflammation in sepsis. Nat Rev Immunol 2006; 6:813–22.

Jiang HL, Xue WJ, Li DQ, Yin AP, et al. Influence of continuous veno-venous hemofiltration on the course of acute pancreatitis. World J Gastroenterol 2005; 21(11):4815–21.

Joannes-Boyau O, Rapaport S, Bazin R, Fleureau C, Janvier G. Impact of high volume hemofiltration on hemodynamic disturbance and outcome during septic shock. ASAIO J 2004; 50:102–9.

Journois D, Israel-Biet P, Rolland B, et al. High-volume, zero-balanced hemofiltration to reduce delayed inflammatory response to cardiopulmonary bypass in children. Anesthesiology 1996; 85:965–76.

Kamijo Y, Soma K, Sugimoto K, et al. The effect of a hemofilter during extracorporeal circulation on hemodynamics in patients with SIRS. Intensive Care Med 2000; 26:1355–9.

Kellum JA, Bellomo R. Hemofiltration in sepsis: where do we go from here? Crit Care 2000; 4:69–71.

Kellum JA, Johnson JP, Kramer D, et al. Diffusive vs. convective therapy: effects on mediators of inflammation in patients with severe systemic inflammatory response syndrome. Crit Care Med 1998; 26:1995–2000.

Kramer P, Wigger W, Rieger J, et al. Arterio-venous hemofiltration: a new simple method of treatment of overhydrated patients resistant to diuretics. Klin Wochenschr 1977; 55:1121–2.

Kumar VA, Yeun JY, Depner TA, et al. Extended daily dialysis vs. continuous hemodialysis for ICU patients with acute renal failure: a two-year single center report. Int J Artif Organs 2004; 27:371–9.

Lee PA, Weger GW, Pryor RW, et al. Effects of filter pore size on efficacy of continuous arteriovenous hemofiltration therapy for Staphylococcus aureus–induced septicemia in immature swine. Crit Care Med 1998; 26:730–7.

Marshall JC. Such stuff as dreams are made on: mediator-directed therapy in sepsis. Nat Rev Drug Discov 2003; 2:391–405.

Mink SN, Li X, Bose D, et al. Early but not delayed continuous arteriovenous hemofiltration improves cardiovascular function in sepsis in dogs. Intensive Care Med 1999; 25:733–43.

Morgera S, Rocktaschel J, Haase M, et al. Intermittent high permeability hemofiltration in septic patients with acute renal failure. Int Care Med 2003; 29:1989–95.

Morgera A, Haase M, Kuss T, et al. Pilot study on the effects of high cutoff hemofiltration on the need for norepinephrine in septic patients with acute renal failure. Crit Care Med 2006; 34:2099–104.

Nadel S, Goldstein B, Williams MD, et al. Drotrecogin alfa (activated) in children with severe sepsis: a multicentre phase III randomised controlled trial. Lancet 2007; 369:836–43.

Nillson A, Fant C, Nyden M, et al. Lipopolysaccharide removal by a peptide-functionalized surface. Colloids Surf Biointerfaces 2005; 40:99–106.

Oudemans-van Straaten HM, Bosman RJ, van der Spoel JI, et al. Outcome of critically ill patients treated with intermittent high-volume haemofiltration: a prospective cohort analysis. Intensive Care Med 1999; 25:814–21.

Page B, Vieillard-Baron A, Chergui K, et al. Early veno-venous haemodiafiltration for sepsis-related multiple organ failure. Crit Care 2005; 9:R755–63.

Peachey TD, Eason JR, Ware RJ, et al. Pump control of continuous arteriovenous haemodialysis. Lancet 1988; 2:878.

Perez XL, Sabater J, Oliver E, et al. Eficacia inicial de dos técnicas de depuración renal en pacientes con shock séptico y fracaso renal agudo. Hemofiltración de Alto Flujo (HVHF) vs coupled plasma filtration adsorption (CPFA). Med Intensiva 2007; 31 (Suppl 1):1–116.

Piccinni P, Dan M, Barbacini S, et al. Early isovolaemic haemofiltration in oliguric patients with septic shock. Intensive Care Med 2006; 32:80–6.

Ratanarat R, Brendolan A, Ricci Z, et al. Pulse high-volume haemofiltration for treatment of severe sepsis: effects on hemodynamics and survival. Crit Care 2005; 9:R294–302.

Reeves JH, Warwick W, Shann F, Layton JE, et al. The plasmafiltration in sepsis study group. Continuous plasmafiltration in sepsis syndrome. Plasmafiltration in Sepsis Study Group. Crit Care Med 1999; 27:2096–104.

Remick DG. Cytokine therapeutics for the treatment of sepsis: why has nothing worked? Curr Pharm Des 2003; 9:75–82.

Remick DG. Pathophysiology of sepsis. Am J Pathol 2007; 170:1435–44.

Remick DG, Kunkel RG, Larrick JW, et al. Acute in vivo effects of human recombinant tumor necrosis factor. Lab Invest 1987; 56:583–90.

Ricc Z, Bonello M, Salvatori G, et al. Continuous renal replacement technology: from adaptive devices to flexible multipurpose machines. Crit Care Resusc 2004; 6:180–7.

Ricci Z, Ronco C, Bachetoni A, et al. Solute removal during continuous renal replacement therapy in critically ill patients: convection versus diffusion. Crit Care 2006; 10:R67.

Rigato O, Salomao R. Impaired production of interferon-gamma and tumor necrosis factor-alpha but not interleukin 10 in whole blood of patients with sepsis. Shock 2003; 19:113–6.

Rogiers P, Zhang H, Smail N, et al. Continuous venovenous hemofiltration improves cardiac performance by mechanisms other than tumor necrosis factor-[alpha] attenuation during endotoxic shock. Crit Care Med 1999; 27:1848–55.

Ronco C, Bellomo R. Dialysis in intensive care unit patients with acute kidney injury: continuous therapy is superior. Clin J Am Soc Nephrol 2007; 2:597–600.

Ronco C, Bellomo R, Homel P, et al. Effects of different doses in continuous veno-venous haemofiltration on outcomes of acute renal failure: a prospective randomised trial. Lancet 2000; 356:26–30.

Ronco C, Ricci Z, Bellomo R. Importance of increased ultrafiltration volume and impact on mortality: sepsis and cytokine story and the role of continuous veno-venous haemofiltration. Curr Opin Nephrol Hypertens 2001; 10:755–61.

Root RK, Lodato RF, Patrick W, et al. Multicenter, double blind, placebo-controlled study of the use of filgastrim in patients hospitalized with pneumonia and severe sepsis. Crit Care Med 2003; 31:367–73.

Sanchez-Izquierdo Riera JA, Perez Vela JL, Lozano Quintana MJ, et al. Cytokines clearance during venovenous hemofiltration in the trauma patient. Am J Kidney Dis 1997; 30:483–8.

Sander A, Armbruster W, Sander B, et al. Hemofiltration increases IL-6 clearance in early systemic inflammatory response syndrome but does not alter IL-6 and TNFα plasma concentrations. Intensive Care Med 1997; 23:878–84.

Saudan P, Niederberger M, De Seigneux S, et al. Adding a dialysis dose to continuous hemofiltration increases survival in patients with acute renal failure. Kidney Int 2006; 70:1312–7.

Schiffl H, Lang SM, König A, et al. Biocompatible membranes in acute renal failure: prospective case controlled study. Lancet 1994; 344:570–2.

Schiffl H, Lang SM, Fischer R. Daily hemodialysis and the outcome of acute renal failure. N Engl J Med 2002; 346:305–10.

Schrier RW, Wang W. Acute renal failure and sepsis. N Engl J Med 2004; 351:159–69.

Stegmayr BG, Banga R, Berggren L, et al. Plasma exchange as rescue therapy in multiple organ failure including acute renal failure. Crit Care Med 2003; 31:1730–6.

Storck M, Hartl WH, Zimme E, et al. Comparison of pump-driven and spontaneous continuous haemofiltration in postoperative acute renal failure. Lancet 1991; 337:452–5.

Tapper H, Herwald H. Modulation of hemostatic mechanisms in bacterial infectious diseases. Blood 2000; 96:2329–37.

Tetta C, Gianotti L, Cavaillon JM, et al. Coupled plasma filtration-adsorption in a rabbit model of endotoxic shock. Crit Care Med 2000; 28:1526–33.

Uchino S, Bellomo R, Goldsmith D, et al. Super high flux hemofiltration: a new technique for cytokine removal. Intensive Care Med 2002; 28:651–5.

Vinsonneau C, Camus C, Combes A, et al. Hemodiafe Study Group: continuous venovenous haemodiafiltration versus intermittent haemodialysis for acute renal failure in patients with multiple-organ dysfunction syndrome: a multicentre randomised trial. Lancet 2006; 368:379–85.

Waage A, Halstensen A, Espevik T. Association between tumour necrosis factor in serum and fatal outcome in patients with meningococcal disease. Lancet 1987; 1:355–7.

Warren BL, Eid A, Singer P, et al. Caring for the critically ill patient. High-dose antithrombin III in severe sepsis: a randomized controlled trial. JAMA 2001; 286:1869–78.

Weksler N, Chorni I, Gurman GM, et al. Continuous venovenous hemofiltration improves intensive care unit, but not hospital survival rate, in nonoliguric septic patients. J Crit Care 2001; 16:69–73.

Yekebas EF, Eisenberger CF, Ohnesorge H, et al. Attenuation of sepsis related immunoparalysis by continuous venovenous hemofiltration in experimental porcine pancreatitis. Crit Care Med 2001; 29:1423–30.

Chapter 7
Optimal Antibiotic Use in Severe Community-Acquired Pneumonia

Alejandro Rodríguez, Mónica Magret, and Jordi Rello

7.1 Introduction

Community-acquired pneumonia (CAP) is the main cause of death due to infectious disease in the developed countries. Although the incidence is not available in most countries, it represents more than 600,000 hospital admissions in the United States (Barlett et al. 2000) and 50,000 in the United Kingdom each year (Hirani and Macfarlane 1997). The cost is higher for nonsurvivors than for survivors (around $7,500 of an in-hospital case) (Fine et al. 1997).

Since the use of penicillin, the mortality rates of severe CAP have not decreased significantly despite advances in antimicrobial therapy and technical improvements in the ICU. Fine et al. (1997) reported that only 10% of hospitalized patients are admitted to ICU, and that the mortality rate in intubated patients reaches 40%. This mortality rate depends on the interaction between the host factors (age, comorbidities, genetic predisposition, and immunocompromise), microorganism characteristics, and optimal antibiotic use (Luján et al. 2006) (Fig. 7.1). In a recent study, Waterer et al. (2001a,b) suggest that CAP patients with septic shock appear to have different genotypes than those with hypoxemic respiratory failure without shock.

The constant increase in the number of elderly and immunocompromised patients (those receiving steroids, organ transplant recipients, HIV patients), the better survival rates of patients affected by chronic illness, and the need for appropriate empirical antibiotics administration are reasons that justify continuing research, focused on improving the diagnosis, defining risk factors that influence outcome, and assessing new therapies.

Usually, at the time of initiation of the empirical antibiotic treatment, the responsible microorganism is not identified. In the last decade, different societies (Infectious Disease Society of America – IDSA, American Thoracic Society – ATS, and British Thoracic Society – BTS) have published guidelines to help physicians in the management of CAP (Barlett et al. 2000; ATS 1993; BTS 2001).

Several studies (Malone and Shaban 2001; Dean et al. 2006; Mortensen et al. 2004) on patients with severe CAP (SCAP) have emphasized the importance of appropriate empirical therapy in reducing disease-related mortality; however, the optimal regimen has not been well defined from large case series. The use of

J. Rello, M.I. Restrepo (eds.) *Sepsis: New Strategies for Management.*
doi:10.1007/978-3-540-79001-3 © Springer-Verlag 2008

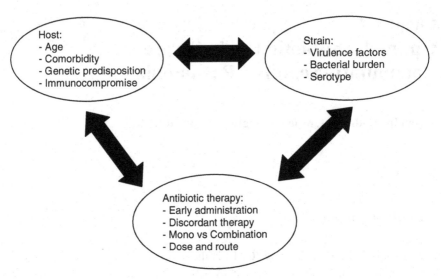

Fig. 7.1 Interaction factors influencing survival in severe community-acquired pneumonia

empiric antimicrobial therapy concordant with international guidelines is associated with decrease mortality among patients with CAP. One study reported a 4.4-fold reduction in mortality if the ATS therapy guidelines were followed (Malone and Shaban 2001). Other authors have observed similar results (Dean et al. 2006; Mortensen et al. 2004). However, these studies have limitations, such as the use of administrative databases, focus on specific patient groups, such as those with bacteremic pneumococcal pneumonia (Waterer et al. 2001a,b; Baddour et al. 2004), or low risk of mortality (Brown et al. 2003). Recently, our group (Bodí et al. 2005) reported the first study to evaluate the impact of the adherence to IDSA guidelines for severe episodes of CAP admitted to ICU. Multivariate analysis found associations between higher mortality rate and age, APACHE II score, immunocompromise, and nonadherence to IDSA guidelines for antibiotic treatment. Interestingly, adherence to IDSA guidelines was the only potentially modifiable factor for improving the prognosis of ICU patients with SCAP.

Considering the few information about treatment of critically ill patients with SCAP, we focused this chapter on the antimicrobial treatment of a subgroup of patients admitted to ICU due to SCAP, specially, on the optimal antibiotic use.

7.2 Antibiotic Therapy: New Concepts

Until now, the in vitro susceptibility of the microorganisms was considered the reference aspect for the antibiotic efficacy for pneumonia (Pea and Viale 2006), and was used to define the concept of "appropriate therapy." Indeed, other factors must be considered to achieve what we call "appropriate," "adequate," or "optimal" antibiotic therapy for pneumonia (Rello and Mallol 2006) (Fig. 7.2). The "appropriate"

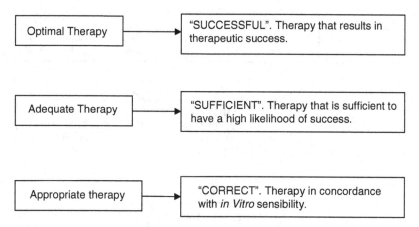

Fig. 7.2 New concepts about antibiotic therapy

or concordant antimicrobial therapy only refers to the in vitro susceptibility. Thus, the main synonym of "appropriate" is "correct." Although fundamental, this might not suffice for the optimal care of critically ill patients. Timely administration of appropriate antimicrobial therapy, particularly in the subset of patients with highest severity, is a crucial factor to improve survival (Houck et al. 2004). In addition, most of the dosing regimens are administered regardless of the infection site and the pathophysiological conditions of the patients. Antibiotic effective concentrations should be guaranteed at the infection site. In critically ill patients, this can be a very difficult goal to achieve considering their complex pathophysiological conditions. Mechanical ventilation increases over 50% the volume of distribution of drugs (Pinder et al. 2002). Thus, higher doses of antimicrobial agents may be required to achieve adequate concentration in the site of infection (Pea and Viale 2006). Therefore, "adequate" antimicrobial therapy should take into account the interaction between the bacterial pathogen and the antimicrobial agent at the minimal inhibitory concentration (MIC). Adequate antibiotic therapy would be the prescription that is sufficient to have a high likelihood of success, beyond the "appropriateness" of the choice. Finally, "optimal" therapy for pneumonia should consider additional factors in addition to the in vitro susceptibility and the penetration into the infectious site, like the anti-inflammatory effects of antibiotics. Thus, "optimal" therapy is that one that results in therapeutic success (Pea and Viale 2006; Rello and Mallol 2006; Wunderink 2004) (Fig. 7.3).

7.3 Management of SCAP

The adequate management of SCAP includes the appropriate antibiotic treatment, management of septic shock, control of the inflammatory response, and ventilatory support. However, in this chapter we will focus only on antibiotic treatment.

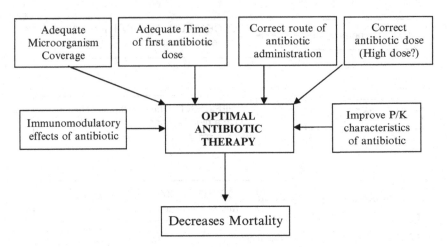

Fig. 7.3 Optimal antibiotic therapy (modified from Pea and Viale 2006)

7.3.1 Antibiotic Treatment

Several studies have demonstrated that an inadequate empiric antibiotic treatment is associated with a significant increase in mortality (Pachón et al. 1990; Torres et al. 1991; Rello et al. 2006; Niederman et al. 1993; Gordon et al. 1996). Inadequate antibiotic treatment is defined as the therapy administered during the first two days of pneumonia onset, which is inactive (intermediate or resistant) in vitro to the responsible microorganism (Luján et al. 2006).

In most cases, the antibiotic treatment begins in an empiric way, covering the most frequent microorganism and considering the risk factors of each patient. However, there is no uniformly accepted definition of SCAP. Many studies have described an entity referred to as SCAP, without providing a specific definition, and requiring only that the patients had been admitted to the ICU (Fine et al. 1997; Waterer et al. 2001a,b; Mortensen et al. 2004; Houck et al. 2004). This has led to tremendous variability in both, the patients and the mortality rate described as SCAP. The ATS has attempted to provide a working set of criteria for this illness (Niederman et al. 1993). In their initial statement, SCAP was characterized by the presence of any of the following features: (1) respiratory rate > 30/min; (2) PaO_2/FiO_2 ratio < 250; (3) need for mechanical ventilation; (4) bilateral, multilobar, or rapidly expanding infiltrates; (5) shock, and (6) oliguria or acute renal failure. However, 65% of all patients admitted to the hospital had at least one of the severe pneumonia features (Gordon et al. 1996). Thus, we still need a more specific definition that better defines a population needing ICU admission for SCAP. We believe that probably patients having shock or needing mechanical ventilation fit in the best definition of SCAP, and these ICU admission criteria have been considered in recent IDSA/ATS guidelines (Mandell et al. 2007).

A major goal of therapy is the eradication of the infecting organism, with resultant resolution of the clinical disease. Appropriate drug selections dependent on the causative microorganism and its antibiotic susceptibility. Acute pneumonia can be caused by a wide variety of pathogens. However, *Streptococcus pneumoniae, Legionella sp.*, and *Haemophilus influenzae* are the main pathogens to cover (Bodí et al. 2005). Until more accurate and rapid diagnostic methods are available, the initial treatments for most patients remain empirical and physicians should consider specific risk factors for each patient (gram-negative pathogens) (Rello et al. 1996, 2003). Recently, in the community setting have appeared methicilin-resistant *Staphylococcus aureus* (MRSA) as severe pulmonary infections (pneumonia or empyema) (Kollef and Micek 2006). At difference to healthcare-associated MRSA, community-acquired MRSA is more susceptible to a wider class of antibiotics but it continues being more virulent, since it usually produces the Panton-Valentine leukocidin (PVL) that makes necrotizing pneumonia. At this time, in contrast to the observed one in America, the community-MRSA is not a frequent pathogen isolated in Europe.

S. pneumoniae is the most frequent microorganism in SCAP. Interestingly, a higher mortality rate for CAP patients has not been reported from countries with high levels of in vitro resistance for *S.pneumoniae* compared with those with lower resistance rates (Lode et al. 2003). Therefore, it is important to emphasize that in vitro resistance may not have the anticipated impact on the outcome.

The most recent IDSA/ATS Guidelines (Mandell et al. 2007) recommend for patients admitted to ICU to begin with a wide spectrum antibiotic treatment. The combination therapy with two different antibiotics that include a potent antipneumococcal β-lactam (cefotaxime, ceftriaxone, or ampicillin-sulbactam) plus a macrolide (level II evidence) or a respiratory fluoroquinolone (level I evidence) is the treatment suggested for critically ill patients. Because septic shock and mechanical ventilation are the clearest reasons for ICU admission, the majority of ICU patients would still require dual therapy. However, these recommendations were not obtained from clinical trials and have been extrapolated from nonsevere cases, in conjunction with case series and retrospective analyses of cohorts with SCAP (Mandell et al. 2007). In fact, many of these trials involved a discretionary use of antibiotic and most were pharmaceutical trials that deliberately excluded ICU patients. Thus, the implications of empirical antibiotic therapy for ICU patients with severe CAP remain unknown.

7.3.2 Mono- or Combination Therapy

Only 20% of CAP patients require hospitalization, and the mortality rate is lower than 10%, regardless of the antibiotic regimen received. Up to 10% of all hospitalized patients with CAP are finally admitted to ICU. This group of patients represents only a small fraction of all of the CAP cases, but in terms of mortality, it is the most important strata.

In the last ten years, many different studies have evaluated the impact of the dual antibiotic treatment for SCAP on mortality. These retrospective and observational studies (Waterer et al. 2001a,b; Baddour et al. 2004) have showed higher rates of survival in patients who are treated with a combination antibiotic therapy. However, the studied population included patients with pneumococcal bacteremic CAP and their conclusions might not be extrapolated to the treatment of all patients with SCAP. Three of these retrospective studies (Waterer et al. 2001a,b; Baddour et al. 2004; Martínez et al. 2003) reported that the benefit was higher in patients with SCAP who received a combination therapy. Indeed, Waterer et al. (2001a,b) observed an 11.3% absolute mortality difference (18.2% vs. 6.9%, $p = 0.02$) favoring the dual therapy. After controlling for comorbidities and the APACHE II score predicted mortality, there was a 6.4-times increased risk of death associated with monotherapy (95% CI 1.9–21.7). However, all deaths occurred in patients with a PSI score over 90, and therefore there was no mortality difference between antibiotic strategies in milder disease. In addition, Baddour et al. (2004) reported that there was a substantial 14-day survival advantage in favor of the combination therapy when the analysis was restricted to patients with severe disease (23.4% vs. 55.3%, $p = 0.001$). Finally, Martínez JA et al. (2003) examined 409 patients with bacteremic pneumococcal pneumonia. The authors evaluated the outcome of patients according to the use of monotherapy with a β-lactam or combination therapy with a β-lactam plus a macrolide. After a stepwise logistic regression analysis, shock, age > 65 years, infection with resistant pathogens, and dual therapy were associated with mortality. The association between initial combination therapy and a lower in-hospital mortality rate remained significant after the exclusion of patients who died ≤ 48 h after admission (OR= 0.4, CI 0.17–0.92).

Although the consistent findings of these studies are very suggestive, they all suffer from one or more significant limitations, predominantly arising from the retrospective nature and the special population considered. The lack of controlled trial data in SCAP admitted to ICU is also a problem with respect to the assessment of the impact of antibiotic therapy on survival according to different levels of illness. Recently, Rodríguez et al. (2007) have shown, in a secondary analysis of a prospective multicenter and observational cohort study including 529 ICU patients with SCAP, that the adjusted 28-day in-ICU mortality was similar ($p = 0.99$) for the combination antibiotic therapy and the monotherapy in the absence of shock. On the other hand, in patients with shock, combination antibiotic therapy was associated with significantly higher 28-day adjusted in-ICU survival (hazard ratio= 1.69; 95% CI 1.09–2.6; $p = 0.01$). These data suggest that ICU patients at higher risk of death (in shock) will derive greater benefit from therapeutic interventions focusing survival (Rello and Rodríguez 2003). On the other hand, this finding strongly suggests that combination therapy does not increase ICU survival in CAP patients with lower risk of death (without shock). Thus, the potential benefits of combination therapy may be limited to the most severely ill patients.

The impact of the combination therapy on mortality in critically ill patients with SCAP is still debated by some investigators questioning whether dual therapy contributes to an improved survival, or if they are secondary to benefit from aggressive initial therapy (Hook et al. 1983), or conversely monotherapy could be indicative of other limitation being placed on treatment. The benefit of combination therapy may be due to: (a) the presence of undetected copathogens, as atypical bacteria, (b) antibiotic synergy, or (c) immunomodulatory effects of macrolides or fluoroquinolones.

Suggested antibiotic regimens for inpatients include a β-lactam combined with a macrolide or monotherapy with a respiratory fluoroquinolone (Mandell et al. 2007). Although *S. pneumoniae* remains to be the leading pathogen in CAP, the rationale for a macrolide supplement or fluoroquinolone monotherapy lies in its ability to cover intracellular (atypical) pathogens as *Legionella pneumophila; Chlamydia pneumoniae, and Mycoplasma pneumoniae*. However, only coverage for *L. pneumophila* is recommended for patients in intensive care units.

Controversy still exists in the literature regarding the need to use antimicrobials covering atypical pathogens when initially treating hospitalized CAP patients. A recent international multicenter study (Arnold et al. 2007) observed a significant global presence (about 20%) of atypical pathogens in CAP. The authors reported that patients treated with atypical coverage had lower time to clinical stability (3.2 days vs. 3.7 days, $p < 0.001$), lower length of stay (6.1 days vs. 7.1 days, $p < 0.01$) and lower CAP-related mortality (3.8% vs. 6.4%, $p = 0.05$). However, since few patients required admission to ICU, the role of atypical microorganisms (different to *L. pneumophila)* in ICU patients with CAP remains unknown. In contrast, a meta-analysis (Shefet et al. 2005) found no difference in mortality between regimens with coverage of atypical pathogens and regimens without such a coverage, persisting in all subgroup analysis. In addition, there was a nonsignificant trend toward clinical success when covering the atypical pathogens, but this advantage disappeared when they evaluated high quality methodological studies alone.

The studies, which documented polymicrobial CAP, rely primarily on serologic conversion to diagnose atypical microorganisms, and no such search for atypical pathogens. Waterer et al. (2001a,b) observed that the coverage of these microorganisms did not contribute to the apparent benefit of dual therapy after the multivariate analysis. Our findings (Bodi et al. 2005) agree with the study of Mundy et al. (1998) who observed infrequent identification of atypical pathogens in a prospective series of patients hospitalized at the Johns Hopkins. Thus, the impact of the atypical pathogens in critically ill patients in SCAP seems to be scarce.

Although appealing, the possibility that the antibiotic combination had a synergistic effect on killing activity is difficult to support. There is certainly no data suggesting synergic activity of β-lactams and macrolides. In fact, there is good evidence that no such synergy exists for either cephalosporin/macrolide (Lin 2003) or penicillin/macrolide (Deshpande 2003) combination against *S. pneumoniae*. Thus, ICU patients with SCAP should receive a combination antibiotic therapy with β-lactam and macrolide or fluoroquinolone only to cover *Legionella pneumophila*.

Other possibility is the immunomodulatory effect of the macrolide or fluoroquinolone that is independent of their antibacterial activity. Although fluoroquinolones exhibit some immunomodulatory effects, it is the macrolides that have been most investigated. Experimental and clinical data on the anti-inflammatory effects of macrolides was recently reported (Waterer et al. 2001a,b; Lode et al. 2003; Schultz et al. 1998). Macrolides have shown to reduce the tumor necrosis factor (TNF) and IL-6 production by whole blood after stimuli with heat-killed pneumococci (Schultz et al. 1998). In addition, macrolides appear to enhance polimorphonuclear activity against pneumococci even when the isolates are macrolide resistant, (Cuffini et al. 2002) and to reduce the IgG-mediated lung damage in rats, again probably by the reduction in both TNF and IL-1β release from the alveolar macrophages (Tamaoki et al. 1999). It is worth noting that macrolides have become widely used in panbronchiolitis and cystic fibrosis with their efficacy attributed to immunomodulation rather than antibacterial effects (Schultz 2004). All fluoroquinolones modestly impair rat macrophage chemotaxis (Labro 2000) and transendothelial neutrophil and monocyte migration (Uriarte et al. 2004). However, only moxifloxacin and gatifloxacin inhibited IL-8 production. These actions on endothelial cells may contribute to the inhibitory effects of fluoroquinolones seen in experimental sepsis models, but their clinical relevance is uncertain (Parnham 2005).

The controversy about which is the best dual therapy for SCAP treatment remains unresolved. Several studies (Waterer et al. 2001a,b; Baddour et al. 2004; Martínez et al. 2003) have found that the use of a β-lactam plus a macrolide is associated with significantly lower mortality. Conversely, few studies have examined the combination of β-lactam with fluoroquinolones versus other combination therapies. A recent study (Mortensen et al. 2006) observed that the empiric use of a β-lactam plus a fluoroquinolone was associated with higher 30-day mortality when compared to other guideline-concordant regimes for patients hospitalized with SCAP. This study has the common limitations of observational and retrospective analysis. However, it is in accordance with a recent study of Metersky et al. (2007) who studied the relationship between the initial antibiotic regimen and mortality in a large cohort of Medicare beneficiaries who were hospitalized with bacteremic pneumonia. These authors observed that, compared to patients who received no atypical coverage, patients treated with a macrolide had a lower risk of adjusted in-hospital mortality (OR = 0.59, 95% CI 0.40–0.88; $p = 0.01$) and of 30-day mortality (OR = 0.61, 95% CI 0.43–0.87; $p = 0.007$). Interestingly, there were no significant associations between fluoroquinolones and patients outcome (OR = 0.94, 95% CI 0.69–1.28). Conversely, other studies (Gleason et al. 1999; Burgess and Lewis 2000) found no significant differences between the use of this combination and others. Nevertheless, the mortality rate observed in these trials is much lower than the mortality rate reported for CAP critically ill patients, and it is possible that the patients included in these trials are different from those included in observational studies. Since most studies showing the importance of adding a macrolide to a β-lactam regimen for SCAP are retrospective, only a prospective randomized double-blind trial will resolve whether combination therapy is truly more effective than monotherapy for SCAP. The strength of the association demonstrated in clinical trials provides significant justification to suggest that combination therapy with a macrolide should be the first line option of antibiotic treatment for ICU patients with SCAP.

Finally, in patients with certain risk factors like severe structural lung disease (bronchiectasias), recent antibiotic exposure, or recent hospitalization, P. aeruginosa can be present in the setting of SCAP (Barlett et al. 2000). Rello et al. (2003), in a recent study, have shown that patients with SCAP who need intubation have a significant risk of *Pseudomonas aeruginosa* or *Legionella* infection. Recently, Bodí et al. (2005) showed that COPD, malignancy, and rapid X-ray spread were factors associated with severe pneumonia by *P.aeruginosa*. Due to all of these findings and the high mortality rate of *P.aeruginosa* pneumonia, in all intubated patients with SCAP and risk factors (COPD, malignancy, previous antibiotic therapy, or rapid X-ray spread), we recommend empirical initial antibiotic treatment with two antipseudomonal agents. However, this initial antibiotic treatment should provide appropriate coverage to penicillin-resistant *Streptococcus pneumoniae* and *Legionella spp.*, the most frequent pathogens observed in CAP.

References

American Thoracic Society. Guidelines for the initial management of adults with community-acquired pneumonia: diagnosis, assessment of severity an initial antimicrobial therapy. Am Rev Respir Dis 1993;148:1418–1426.

Arnold FW, Summersgill JT, Lajoie AS, et al. A worldwide perspective of atypical pathogens in community-acquired pneumonia. Am J Respir Crit Care Med 2007;175:1086–1093.

Baddour LM, Yu VL, Klugman KP, et al. Combinations antibiotic therapy lowers mortality among severely ill patients with pneumoccocal bacteriemia. Am J Respir Crit Care Med 2004;170:440–444.

Barlett JG, Dowell SF, Mandell LA, et al. Practice guidelines for the management of community-acquired pneumonia in adults. Clin Infect Dis 2000;31:347–382.

Bodí M, Rodríguez A, Solé-Violan, et al. Antibiotic prescription for community-acquired pneumonia in the intensive care unit: impact of adherence to Infectious Diseases Society of America Guidelines on survival. Clin Infect Dis 2005;41:1709–1716.

British Thoracic Society. BTS guidelines for the management of community-acquired pneumonia in adults. Thorax 2001;56:iv1–iv64.

Brown RB, Iannini P, Gross P, et al. Impact of antibiotic choice on clinical outcomes in community-acquired pneumonia. Chest 2003;123:1503–1511.

Burgess DS, Lewis JS. Effect of macrolides as part of initial empiric therapy on medical outcomes for hospitalized patients with community-acquired pneumonia. Clin Ther 2000;22:872–878.

Cuffini AM, Tullio V, Mandras N, et al. Clarithromycin mediated the expression of polimorphonu-clear granulocyte response against *Streptocuccus pneumoniae* strains with different patterns of susceptibility and resistance to penicillin and clarithromycin. Int J Tissue React 2002;24:37–44.

Dean NC, Bateman KA, Donnelly SM, et al. Improved clinical outcome with utilization of a community-acquired pneumonia guideline. Chest 2006;130:794–799.

Deshpande LM. Jr. Antagonism between penicillin and erythromycin against *Streptococcus pneumoniae*: does it exist? Diagn Microbiol Infect Dis 2003;46:223–225.

Fine MJ, Auble TE, Yealy DM, et al. A prediction rule to identify low-risk patients with community-acquired pneumonia. N Engl J Med 1997;336:243–250.

Gleason PP, Meehan TP, Fine JM, et al. Association between initial antimicrobial therapy and medical outcomes for hospitalized elderly patients with pneumonia. Arch Intern Med 1999;159:2562–2572.

Gordon G, Throop D, Berberian L, et al. Validation of ATS guidelines for community-acquired pneumonia in hospitalized patients. Am J Respir Crit Care Med 1996;153:A257.

Hirani NA, Macfarlane JT. Impact of management guidelines on the outcome of severe community-acquired pneumonia. Thorax 1997;52:17–21.

Hook EW, Horton CA, Schaberg DR. Failure of intensive care unit support to influence mortality from pneumococcal bacteremia. JAMA 1983;249:1055–1057.

Houck PM, Bratzler DW, Nsa W, et al. Timing of antibiotic administration and outcomes for medicare patients hospitalized with community-acquired pneumonia. Arch Intern Med 2004;164:637–644.

Kollef MH, Micek ST. Methicillin-resistant Staphylococcus aureus: a new community-acquired pathogen? Curr Opin Infect Dis 2006;19:161–168.

Labro MT. Interference of antibacterial agents with phagocytic functions: immunomodulation or "immuno-fairy tales"? Clin Microbiol Rev 2000;13:615–650.

Lin E. Lack of synergy of erythromycin combined with penicillin or cefotaxime against Streptococcus pneumoniae in vitro. Antimicrob Agents Chemother 2003;47:1151–1153.

Lode H, Grossman C, Choudhri S, et al. Sequential IV/PO moxifloxacin treatment of patients with severe community-acquired pneumonia. Respir Med 2003;97:1134.

Luján M, Gallego M, Rello J. Optimal therapy for severe pneumococcal community-acquired pneumonia. Intensive Care Med 2006;32:971–980.

Malone DC, Shaban HM. Adherence to ATS guidelines for hospitalized patients with community-acquired pneumonia. Ann Pharmacother 2001;35:1180–1185.

Mandell LA, Wunderink RG, Anzueto A, et al. Infectious Disease Society of America/American Thoracic Society Consensus Guidelines on the management of community-acquired pneumonia in adults. Clin Infect Dis 2007;44:S27–S72.

Martínez JA, Horcajada JP, Almela M, et al. Addition of macrolide to a β-lactam-based empirical antibiotic regimen is associated with lower in-hospital mortality for patients with bacteremic pneumococcal pneumonia. Clin Infect Dis 2003;36:389–395.

Metersky ML, Ma A, Houck PM, Bratzler DW. Antibiotic for bacteremic pneumonia: improved outcome with macrolide but not fluoroquinolones. Chest 2007;131:466–473.

Mortensen EM, Restrepo M, Anzueto A, Pugh J. Effects of guideline-concordant antimicrobial therapy on mortality among patients with community-acquired pneumonia. Am J Med 2004;117:726–731.

Mortensen EM, Restrepo I, Anzueto A, Pugh J. The impact of empiric antimicrobial therapy with a β-lactam and fluoroquinolone on mortality for patients hospitalized with severe pneumonia. Crit Care 2006;10:R8.

Mundy LM, Oldach D, Auwaerter PG, et al. Implications for macrolide treatment in community-acquired pneumonia. Chest 1998;113:1201–1206.

Niederman MS, Bass JB, Campbell GD, et al. Guidelines for the initial management of adults with community-acquired pneumonia: diagnosis, assessment of severity and initial antimicrobial therapy. Am Rev Respir Dis 1993;148:1418–1426.

Pachón J, Prado MD, Capote F, et al. Severe community-acquired pneumonia. Etiology, prognosis and treatment. Am Rev Respir Dis 1990;142:369–373.

Parnham MJ. Immunomodulatory effects of antimicrobials in the therapy of respiratory tract infections. Curr Opin Infect Dis 2005;18:125–131.

Pea F, Viale P. The antimicrobial therapy puzzle: could pharmacokinetic-pharmacodynamic relationship be helpful in addressing the issue of appropriate pneumonia treatment in critically ill patients? Clin Infect Dis 2006;42:1764–1471.

Pinder M, Bellomo R, Lipman J. Pharmacological principles of antibiotic prescription in the critically ill. Anaesth Intensive Care 2002;30:134–144.

Rello J, Mallol J. Optimal therapy for methicillin-resistant Staphylococcus aureus pneumonia. What is the best dosing regimen? Chest 2006;130:938–940.

Rello J, Rodriguez A. Improving survival for sepsis: on the cutting edge. Crit Care Med 2003;31:2807–2808.

Rello J, Rodríguez R, Jubert P, et al. Severe community-acquired pneumonia in the elderly: epidemiology and prognosis. Clin Infect Dis 1996;23:723–728.

Rello J, Bodí M, Mariscal D, et al. Microbiogical testing and outcome of patients with severe community-acquired pneumonia. Chest 2003;123:174–180.

Rello J, Rodríguez A, Torres A. Implications on COPD in patients admitted to the ICU by community-acquired pneumonia. A comparison with a cohort of non-COPD patients. Eur Respir J 2006;26:1210–1216.

Rodríguez A, Mendia A, Sirvent JM. Combination antibiotic therapy improves survival in patients with community-acquired pneumonia and shock. Crit Care Med 2007;35:1493–1499.

Schultz MU. Macrolide activities beyond their antimicrobial effects: macrolides in diffuse panbronchiolitis and cystic fibrosis. J Antimicrob Chemother 2004;54:21–28.

Schultz MJ, Speerlman P, Zaat S, et al. Erythromycin inhibits tumor necrosis factor alpha and interleukin 6 production induced by heat-killed *Streptocuccus pneumoniae* in whole blood. Antimicrob Agents Chemother 1998;42:1605–1609.

Shefet D, Robenshtok E, Mical P, Leibovici L. Empirical atypical coverage for inpatients with community-acquired pneumonia. Systematic review of randomized controlled trials. Arch Intern Med 2005;165:1992–2000.

Tamaoki J, Kondo M, Kohri K, et al. Macrolide antibiotics protect against immune complex-induced lung injury in rats: role of nitric oxide form alveolar macrophages. J. Immunol 1999;163:2909–2915.

Torres A, Serra-Batlles J, Ferrer A, et al. Severe community-acquired pneumonia. Epidemiology and prognosis factors. Am Rev Respir Dis 1991;114:312–318.

Uriarte SM, Molestina RE, Miller RD, et al. Effects of fluoroquinolones on the migration of human phagocytes through *Chlamydia pneumoniae*-infected and tumor necrosis factor alpha-stimulated endothelial cells. Antimicrob Agents Chemother 2004;48:2538–2543.

Waterer GW, Quasney MW, Cantor RM, et al. Septic shock and respiratory failure in community-acquired pneumonia have different TNF polymorphism associations. Am J Respir Crit Care Med 2001a;163:1599–1604.

Waterer GW, Somes GW, Wunderink RG. Monotherapy may be suboptimal for severe bacteriemic pneumococcal pneumonia. Arch Intern Med 2001b;161:1837–1842.

Wunderink RG. A long and winding road. Crit Care Med 2004;32:1077–1079.

Chapter 8
Dose Adjustment and Pharmacodynamic Considerations for Antibiotics in Severe Sepsis and Septic Shock

Andrew Udy, Jason Roberts, Robert Boots, and Jeffrey Lipman

8.1 Introduction

Prescription of antibiotics in the critically ill is a complex process. It requires consideration of the likely causative organism/s, an appreciation of the underlying pathophysiological state and how this dynamic process influences drug distribution, metabolism and elimination. Associated organ dysfunction, fluid shifts and altered immune status are common, and each can influence the efficacy of many antimicrobial agents. This chapter will focus on the prescription of antibiotics commonly used in the treatment of critically ill patients with severe sepsis or septic shock. Early appropriate antimicrobial therapy remains the cornerstone of successful treatment in this group (Kollef et al. 1999; Ibrahim et al. 2000; Garnacho-Montero et al. 2003; Valles et al. 2003). Pharmacokinetic and pharmacodynamic principles will be reviewed, with the aim to optimize dosing and improve outcome. There are similar considerations concerning the use of antifungal and possibly antiviral agents in the critically ill; however, a wider discussion of these agents is beyond the scope of this chapter.

8.2 Applied Clinical Pharmacology

Successful treatment of an infection involves optimizing the interaction between the host, the pathogen and the antibiotic (Nicolau 1998). Recommended antibiotic regimens have often been derived from studies on healthy volunteers or non-critically ill patient groups, making extrapolation to dosing in severe sepsis difficult. Key considerations involve a variety of pathophysiological changes associated with sepsis, and their effects on the pharmacokinetic and pharmacodynamic parameters of the chosen antibiotic. This process is dynamic, and ongoing evaluation of illness severity, organ function and the resuscitation status are necessary to allow the timely adjustment of antibiotic dosing.

J. Rello, M.I. Restrepo (eds.) *Sepsis: New Strategies for Management.*   97
doi:10.1007/978-3-540-79001-3 © Springer-Verlag 2008

8.2.1   Pharmacokinetic Considerations

Pharmacokinetics (PK) refers to the study of changes in drug concentration over time. The primary PK parameters of importance to antibiotics include:

- *Volume of distribution (Vd).* Apparent (hypothetical) volume of fluid that contains the total amount of administered drug, at the same concentration as that measured in plasma.
- *Clearance (CL).* Volume of plasma effectively cleared of the drug per unit time. Total clearance is the sum of the clearances for each eliminating organ or tissue.
- *Plasma half-life ($T_{1/2}$).* Time required to decrease the plasma concentration by one half.
- C_{max}. The peak concentration achieved by a single dose.
- C_{min}. The lowest concentration during a dosing period.
- *Area under the curve (AUC).* The area under the plasma concentration–time curve.

Antibiotics can be classified by their affinity for water (hydrophilic) or lipids (lipophilic). Where hydrophilic drugs are typically distributed in extracellular water, lipophilic drugs may distribute intracellularly and into body fat, favouring bioaccumulation. Protein binding of antibiotics either to albumin or alpha-1 acid glycoprotein (AAG) effects their distribution throughout the body and their biological effect. More highly bound drugs generally have a longer duration of action and a lower volume of distribution. The free drug concentration is important for clinical effect, and is influenced by plasma protein levels and binding competition from other drugs. Consideration of these basic pharmacokinetic factors can be used to determine whether appropriate concentrations of the antibiotic are being delivered to the target area (Nicolau 2003).

8.2.2   Pharmacodynamic Considerations

The pharmacodynamic (PD) effect of antibiotics refers to the ability of the antibiotic to kill or inhibit the growth of the infective organism. How this is effected by an antibiotic's PK properties is referred to as "pharmacokinetics-pharmacodynamics or PK–PD characteristics" but will be termed "pharmacodynamics" (PD) here. PD parameters include:

- *T > MIC.* The time for which a drug's concentration remains above the minimum inhibitory concentration (MIC) for bacterial growth during a given dosing period
- C_{max}/MIC. The ratio of the maximum antibiotic concentration (C_{max}) to the MIC of the pathogen
- $AUC_{0–24}/MIC$. The ratio of the area under the concentration time curve during a 24-hour time period to the MIC of the pathogen (see Fig. 8.1)

Pharmacodynamically, the rate and extent of an antibiotic's bactericidal activity is dependent on the interaction between drug concentrations at the site of infection, bacterial load, phase of bacterial growth and the MIC for the pathogen (Nicolau 2003). It follows that a change in any of these factors will affect the PD profile of the antibiotic against a particular pathogen and may affect the outcome of therapy.

8.3   Kill Characteristics of Different Antibiotic Classes

Different antibiotic classes can be generally classified by their bacterial killing characteristics: concentration-dependent killing and time-dependent killing (Fig. 8.1 and Table 8.1). An understanding of these PD properties should be considered for appropriate dose adjustment in individual patients.

These kill characteristics have been determined from in vitro and ex vivo studies and describe the PK measurements that represent optimal bactericidal activity (Nicolau 2003). The β-lactam group of antibiotics have a time-dependent kill characteristic, and as such T > MIC is the best predictor of antibiotic efficacy (Nuytinck et al. 1988; Craig 1998). Maintaining adequate plasma concentrations throughout the dosing interval is essential. In contrast, aminoglycosides have a concentration-dependent (or time-independent) kill characteristic where effect is determined by C_{max}/MIC (Craig 1984; Schentag et al. 1984; Vogelman and Craig 1985, 1986; Moore et al. 1987; Vogelman et al. 1988; Leggett et al. 1989; Roosendaal et al. 1989; Bakker-Woudenberg and Roosendaal 1990; Bouvier d'Yvoire and Maire 1996; Mouton and Vinks 2005). The higher the peak concentration achieved above the MIC, the greater will be the bacterial kill. Fluoroquinolones are more complex, being initially reported to be C_{max}/MIC dependent, although subsequent studies have also found that AUC_{0-24}/MIC is important (Forrest et al. 1993; Gunderson et al. 2001). The pharmacodynamic parameters associated with efficacy for other antibiotics are described in Table 8.1.

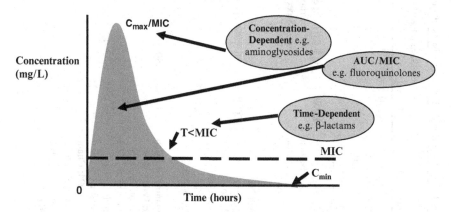

Fig. 8.1 Pharmacokinetic and pharmacodynamic parameters of antibiotics on a concentration vs. time curve

Table 8.1 General PK and PD characteristics of various antibiotics

Antibiotic	Vd (L/kg)	Serum half-life ($T_{1/2}$, h)	Protein binding	Clearance	Post-antibiotic effect	Kill characteristic	PD parameter	Tissue penetration
Aminoglycosides (Mangione and Schentag 1980; Pharmacia Australia 2005)	0.2–0.3	2–3	Low	Renal (Chambers and Sande 1996)	Yes	Concentration dependent	C_{max}/MIC	Poor
β-lactams (Swabb et al. 1983; Barbhaiya et al. 1992; Lipman et al. 1999a, 2001, 2003; Levitt 2003)	ECW	0.5–2 h (longer for ceftriaxone (Stoeckel 1981))	Low (except ceftriaxone (Stoeckel 1981) and flucloxacillin	Renal (McKindley et al. 1996) (some exceptions)	Gram (+) organisms only	Time dependent	T > MIC	Variable
Carbapenems (Mouton et al. 2000)	ECW	1 h (Ertapenem – 4h)	Low (except Ertapenem)	Renal	Yes	Time dependent (Turnidge 1998b)	T > MIC	Good
Vancomycin (Cunha 1995a)	0.2–1.25	4–6	30–55%	Renal (Rybak 2006)	Yes (MacKenzie and Gould 1993)	Concentration and time dependent	AUC_{24}/MIC	Poor
Teicoplanin (Brogden and Peters 1994; Wilson 2000; Barbot et al. 2003)	0.9–1.6	80–160	90%	Renal	Yes (MacKenzie and Gould 1993)	Concentration and time dependent	AUC_{24}/MIC	Poor
Quinupristin/dalfopristin (Bernard et al. 1994; Chant and Rybak 1995; MIMS Australia 2005a)	Q = 0.45 D = 0.24	1.3–1.5	Q = 23–32% D = 50–56%	Hepatic	Yes (E. faecium (Aeschlimann and Rybak 1998) & S. aureus (Griswold et al. 1996))	Concentration dependent	AUC_{24}/MIC	Poor

Drug								
Daptomycin (Woodworth et al. 1992; Dvorchik et al. 2002, 2003)	0.09	5.8–11.6	92%	Renal	Yes	Concentration dependent	C_{max}/MIC	Poor
Tigecycline (Meagher et al. 2005a,b; Muralidharan et al. 2005; Rubinstein and Vaughan 2005)	7–10	37–66	73–79%	Hepatic	Yes (Projan 2000)	Time dependent	AUC_{24}/MIC	Excellent
Telithromycin (Namour et al. 2002; Gattringer et al. 2004; Kasbekar and Acharya 2005; Nguyen and Chung 2005)	2.7–2.9	10–13	60–70%	Renal	Yes	Concentration dependent (Odenholt et al. 2001; Jacobs et al. 2003)	C_{max}/MIC	Variable
Clindamycin (Fass and Saslaw 1972; DeHaan et al. 1973; Gordon et al. 1973; Mann et al. 1987b; Rovers et al. 1995; Mueller et al. 1999)	0.6–1.2	1.5–5	65–90%	Hepatic	Yes (*B. anthracis*) (Athamna et al. 2004)	Time dependent	T > MIC	Excellent
Linezolid (MacGowan 2003; Stalker et al. 2003; Boselli et al. 2005)	0.5–0.6	3.5–7	31%	Hepatic and renal	Yes (*B. anthracis*) (Athamna et al. 2004)	Time dependent	AUC_{24}/MIC	Good
Ciprofloxacin (MICROMEDEX 1974–2005; Brittain et al. 1985; Bennett et al. 1994)	1.2–2.7	3 (4–5 in the elderly)	20–40%	Hepatic	Yes	Concentration and time dependent	AUC_{24}/MIC	Excellent (Smith et al. 2000)

(continued)

Table 8.1 (continued)

Antibiotic	Vd (L/kg)	Serum half-life ($T_{1/2}$, h)	Protein binding	Clearance	Post-antibiotic effect	Kill characteristic	PD parameter	Tissue penetration
Levofloxacin (Chien et al. 1997, 1998)	0.9–1.36	6–8.9	24–38%	Renal	Yes	Concentration and time dependent	AUC_{24}/MIC	Excellent (Smith et al. 2000)
Moxifloxacin (Chien et al. 1997; Stass et al. 1998; Stass 1999)	2.45–3.6	9.3–15.6	39–52%	Hepatic	Yes	Concentration and time dependent	AUC_{24}/MIC	Excellent (Smith et al. 2000)
Gatifloxacin (MICROMEDEX 1974–2005; Nakashima et al. 1995)	1.98–2.3	6.5–9.6	20%	Hepatic	Yes	Concentration and time dependent	AUC_{24}/MIC	Excellent (Smith et al. 2000)
Azithromycin (Zuckerman 2004; Chiu et al. 2002)	13–31	40–68	7–50%	Hepatic	Yes	Concentration and time dependent	AUC_{24}/MIC	Excellent

ECW extracellular water

8.3.1 Post-antibiotic Effect

Most antibiotics demonstrate a post-antibiotic effect (PAE): the continued suppression of bacterial growth for prolonged periods when drug concentrations fall below the MIC of the bacteria (Rodvold 2001). β-lactams demonstrate a modest PAE against gram-positive organisms but no PAE (except carbapenems) against gram-negative organisms (Bustamante et al. 1984; Tauber et al. 1984; Gudmundsson et al. 1986; Craig and Ebert 1991; Fantin et al. 1991; Craig 1993, 1998; Tessier et al. 1999; Rodvold 2001; Drusano 2004). Aminoglycosides demonstrate a significant PAE (>3h), the duration of which is concentration dependent (Craig 1984; Vogelman and Craig 1985, 1986; Moore et al. 1987; Vogelman et al. 1988; Roosendaal et al. 1989; Bakker-Woudenberg and Roosendaal 1990; Mouton and Vinks 2005). Fluoroquinolones also possess a prolonged PAE (Lode et al. 1998; Turnidge 1998a). Interestingly, the PAE of an agent can change in states of altered immune function, being reduced in neutropenia (Klatersky 1986; Kapusnik et al. 1988; Fisman and Kaye 2000) or in critically ill patients with sepsis. However, this has not been widely characterized for all antibiotics.

8.3.2 Post-β-lactamase Inhibitor Effect

Post-β-lactamase inhibitor effect (PLIE) refers to a period of continued suppression of bacterial growth after removal of a β-lactamase inhibitor (also known as a suicide inhibitor) (Thorburn et al. 1996). It has been shown to occur in vitro for amoxicillin plus clavulanate (Thorburn et al. 1996) and more recently ceftazidime plus sulbactam (Lavigne et al. 2004). This effect may be utilized in treating extended-spectrum β-lactamases (ESBLs), and enable reduced β-lactam doses (Thorburn et al. 1996). However, scarce clinical evidence exists for the clinical relevance of PLIE.

8.3.3 Inoculum Effect

The inoculum effect refers to the activity of certain antibiotics in the presence of a large bacterial load (initially described with E. coli). High bacterial concentrations make third generation β-lactams less effective (Kim 1985), and is thought to be due to the production of β-lactamases (Levison 1995). Broader spectrum β-lactams, including fourth generation cephalosporins have a clinical advantage in this respect (Phelps et al. 1986; Hoepelman et al. 1993; Jauregui et al. 1993). In clinical practice, the identification of bacterial load is difficult and thus dose changes on the basis of these observations are not indicated at this time. However, this does underscore the importance of early effective broad-spectrum antibiotic therapy in the critically ill.

8.4   Sepsis

While a definition and conceptual framework for sepsis is continuing to evolve, the process is most widely thought of as a systemic inflammatory response syndrome (SIRS) triggered by an overwhelming infection (Bone et al. 1992; Calandra and Cohen 2005). Severe sepsis occurs upon failure or dysfunction of at least one organ, and septic shock is defined by hypotension in the setting of severe sepsis, unresponsive to fluid resuscitation. The pathogenesis of sepsis is complex (Parrillo 1993; Grocott-Mason and Shah 1998; Calandra and Cohen 2005; Rice and Bernard 2005), and research in this area is an ongoing process. While much effort has been directed at cellular and humoral targets to limit the associated inflammatory and coagulation cascades (Rice and Bernard 2005), none of these interventions have been found to be as important or effective as optimal early antibiotic therapy (Kollef et al. 1999; Garnacho-Montero et al. 2003; Harbarth et al. 2003; Hugonnet et al. 2003; MacArthur et al. 2004; Rice and Bernard 2005; Kumar et al. 2006). The host's recognition of and response to the invading microorganism largely determine the degree of pathophysiological disturbance and clinical sequelae. Therefore, knowledge of the pathophysiological and pharmacokinetic changes in sepsis are necessary to ensure optimal prescription of antibiotics (Kieft et al. 1993; Joukhadar et al. 2001).

8.4.1   Pathophysiological Changes in Sepsis that can Affect Pharmacokinetics

Figure 8.2 schematically depicts the pharmacokinetic changes that can occur due to the altered pathophysiology during sepsis.

8.4.1.1   Altered Capillary Permeability

Endotoxins from bacteria or fungi can stimulate the production of a variety of endogenous mediators (van der Poll 2001), which may effect the vascular endothelium directly or indirectly. This can result in either vasoconstriction or vasodilatation with altered distribution of blood flow, endothelial damage and increased capillary permeability. This capillary leak syndrome results in fluid shifts from the intravascular compartment to the interstitial space (Nuytinck et al. 1988; Gosling et al. 1994) known as "third spacing". For water-soluble drugs, this will result in an increase in Vd, decreasing the plasma concentration. It is uncommon for the Vd of lipophilic agents to be affected by "third spacing".

8.4.1.2   Hypoalbuminaemia

Hypoalbuminaemia is a frequently encountered problem in the critically ill. It may develop de novo in severe sepsis as a consequence of increased protein capillary leak, fluid loading, increased catabolism and under-feeding. A low plasma albumin

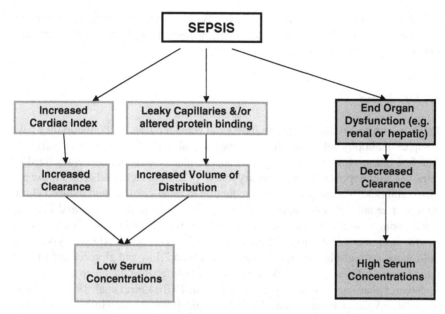

Fig. 8.2 Basic pathophysiological changes that can occur during sepsis and their subsequent pharmacokinetic effect

concentration results in a reduction in oncotic pressure and encourages fluid extravasation and interstitial oedema formation. This will increase the Vd of hydrophilic antibiotics such as aminoglycosides. The Vd will also be increased for agents that are highly albumin bound and renally excreted (e.g. ceftriaxone and teicoplanin), resulting in a greater free-fraction of drug and higher renal clearances (Rowland 1990; Pea and Furlanut 2001; Barbot et al. 2003).

Recent work in critically ill patients with severe sepsis treated with 2-g IV ceftri-axone (protein binding ~ 90%) once daily has demonstrated an increase in Vd and an almost doubling of drug clearance in those patients with normal renal function but severe hypoalbuminaemia (Joynt et al. 2001). This implies that in patients with severe hypoalbuminaemia and normal renal function, optimum dosing with ceftriaxone may involve either shortening the dosage interval or administration by continuous infusion (Joynt et al. 2001). An increase in the Vd of amikacin (protein binding ~10%) has also been noted in patients with haematological malignancies and hypoalbuminaemia (Romano et al. 1999). It may also have a role in contributing to low trough levels in critically ill children treated with teicoplanin (Sanchez et al. 1999). In summary, consideration should be given to different dosing regimes for hydrophilic antimicrobials in critically ill patients with severe hypoalbuminaemia, to ensure adequate drug concentrations.

8.4.1.3   Post-surgical Drains

Indwelling surgical drains are a source of hidden drug loss. Patients post major abdominal and thoracic surgery can lose drug via this route (Buijk et al. 2002b), and it may contribute to sub-therapeutic levels of hydrophilic antibiotics. The effect is an increase in Vd and clearance perhaps necessitating higher and/or more frequent doses in these patients.

8.4.1.4 Burns

Patients with severe burns deserve individual consideration. Not only do they have complex pathophysiological changes, they are also prone to recurrent infection. The first phase of the burns injury lasts approximately 48 h and is characterized by intra-vascular hypovolaemia secondary to loss of protein-rich fluid across the capillary membrane. This may result in a reduction in renal pre-load and reduced elimination of renally cleared antibiotics. Increasing interstitial oedema and ongoing fluid loading can result in an increase in the Vd of hydrophilic antibiotics, leading to low plasma concentrations. The second phase is characterized by a hypermetabolic state, with a subsequent increase in renal blood flow and glomerular filtration rate (Lesne-Hulin et al. 1997; Weinbren 1999) lasting several days to weeks.

Several pharmacokinetic studies (Zaske et al. 1976; Loirat et al. 1978; Brater et al. 1986; Walstad et al. 1988; Yoshida et al. 1993; Lesne-Hulin et al. 1997; Weinbren 1999) have shown increased clearance of hydrophilic and moderately lipophilic agents during this second phase. As such, higher doses of aminoglycosides are required in burns patients (Hollingsed et al. 1993), and more frequent dosing of glycopeptides is also advocated (Boucher et al. 1992). Regular measurement of trough concentrations is essential to avoid sub-therapeutic levels (Rice 1992). Further detailed review of pharmacokinetic considerations for different antibiotic agents in burns patients is beyond the scope of this chapter, but given the complex pathophysiological changes that occur, and the wide inter-individual variation, therapeutic drug monitoring (TDM) is recommended in this setting.

8.4.1.5 Creatinine Clearance can be Increased or Decreased

Serum creatinine concentration alone is a poor measure of renal function. In the critically ill population, elevated creatinine clearance has been demonstrated despite a serum value within the normal range (Lipman et al. 2001, 2002). Hypotension is a common clinical manifestation of the inflammatory response associated with sepsis, and initial volume loading with intravenous fluids is a cornerstone of early treatment (Rivers et al. 2001). If hypotension persists, vasoactive agents (some of which may be "inoconstrictors") are often utilized (Dellinger et al. 2008) producing higher than normal cardiac indices in these patients (Parrillo et al. 1990; Parrillo 1993; Pea et al. 2000). In the absence of significant organ dysfunction, this results in increased renal blood flow and higher creatinine and drug clearance (Di Giantomasso et al. 2002, 2003, 2005) and is a major reason to consider modification of drug dose/dosing intervals in the critically ill (Pinder et al. 2002; Lipman et al. 2003).

As sepsis progresses, significant myocardial depression can occur which leads to a decrease in organ perfusion (Parrillo et al. 1990). Myocardial insufficiency and abnormalities of the macrovascular circulation are compounded by failure of the microcirculation. The resultant end-organ cellular injury may progress to multiple organ dysfunction syndrome (MODS) (Marshall 2001). This often includes renal and/or hepatic dysfunction with failure of homeostatic and excretory mechanisms. Drug elimination half-lives can be prolonged and result in increased antibiotic concentrations and/or accumulation of metabolites (Power et al. 1998).

8.4.1.6   Determining Renal Function in Critically Ill Patients with Sepsis

Accurate knowledge of renal function is a critical factor for dosing antibiotics, as most of these agents are eliminated by the kidney. However, assessment of renal function in the critically ill patient with sepsis is not straightforward. Accepted norms for calculating creatinine clearance (as a marker of renal function) in "normal" ward patients, such as the Cockroft-Gault method (Cockroft and Gault 1976), and the Modified Diet in Renal Disease (MDRD) study (Levey et al. 1999) are not accurate in the critically ill (Roberts et al. 2005). As such, the most effective way to calculate renal function remains using either an 8-, 12- or 24-h creatinine clearance collection (Wells and Lipman 1997a,b; Pong et al. 2005), although recent work has suggested a 2-h creatinine clearance may be an adequate substitute (Herrera-Gutierrez et al. 2007). If acute renal failure occurs, such that the patient needs renal replacement therapy (RRT) with either intermittent haemodialysis or continuous renal replacement therapy, further considerations for appropriate antibiotic dosing are introduced.

8.4.1.7   Renal Replacement Therapy

Various methods of RRT are available to remove nitrogenous waste products and fluid, and the subsequent effect on antibacterial pharmacokinetics is complex. A detailed review of this subject is beyond the scope of this chapter, although for RRT, the extent of any direct change in drug clearance has often not been investigated. Metabolic and homeostatic factors that need consideration include changes in total body water, albumin and acute phase protein levels, muscle mass, blood pH, bilirubin concentration, renal, hepatic and cardiac function (Joy et al. 1998a,b). The size of the molecule, degree of protein binding, route of elimination, electrostatic charge and Vd will all influence the potential effects of RRT (Joy et al. 1998a,b; Bugge 2001). Technical factors including the type of filter used, blood flow rate, ultrafiltration rate, use of counter current dialysis and membrane interactions, and whether the dialysis is intermittent or continuous are also important considerations (Freebairn and Lipman 1993a,b; Schetz et al. 1995; Joy et al. 1998a,b; Pinder et al. 2002; Trotman et al. 2005). Often the need for RRT is transient in the septic patient, and as native renal function improves, the challenge for the practising clinician is to adjust doses accordingly to ensure therapeutic drug concentrations.

8.5 Duration of Antibiotic Therapy for Critically Ill Patients with Sepsis

Little data exist to rationally guide the duration of antibiotic treatment in critically ill patients. However, increasing awareness of the risks of prolonged courses of broad spectrum agents has led towards shortening the length of treatment. Most courses of antibiotics in ICU are given for an empirical duration based upon site of infection and pathogen. Some data exist to modify durations based upon clinical response.

The Infectious Disease Society of America (IDSA) guidelines on management of community-acquired pneumonia (CAP) in adults (Bartlett et al. 2000) suggests that length of treatment should be guided by clinical factors, such as response, severity and co-morbidities. Specifically, they note that pneumonia caused by *Streptococcus pneumoniae* should be treated until the patient has been afebrile for at least 72 h. Similar recommendations are made for management of neutropenic patients with cancer based upon duration of fever and neutrophil count (Bartlett et al. 2000). Published guidelines can be consulted when considering other systemic infections (Therapeutic Guidelines Antibiotic 2006).

The Surviving Sepsis Campaign (Dellinger et al. 2008) recently produced updated treatment guidelines for the management of severe sepsis and septic shock. These guidelines recommend a typical seven- to ten-day course of antibiotic therapy that should be guided by microbiological results and clinical response. Importantly, the appropriateness of the anti-infective therapy should be reviewed regularly to ensure adequacy of treatment and allow de-escalation where possible (Dellinger et al. 2008). The pathophysiological sequelae of severe sepsis and septic shock are transient and dynamic in nature, and changes in drug distribution, metabolism and elimination can be expected throughout the patients' course. Although there is little literature to guide specific dosage adjustment in critically unwell patients – particularly for many of the newer antimicrobials – daily review of the appropriateness of antibiotic dosage should be undertaken.

8.6 Implications of Under-dosing in Sepsis

The most important clinical consequence of under-dosing in severe sepsis and septic shock is treatment failure. Effective antibiotic therapy is essential to optimize patient outcome (Cunha 1995b; Kollef et al. 1999; Garnacho-Montero et al. 2003; Harbarth et al. 2003; MacArthur et al. 2004). Developing dosing regimens that maximize the rate of response in patients with sepsis is important for accelerating patient recovery, but also in minimizing the development of antibiotic resistance. Under-dosing with β-lactams may facilitate the development of antibiotic resistance, particularly if plasma concentrations fall below the threshold (MIC) for more than half the dosing interval (Fantin et al. 1994). Inappropriately low dosing of ciprofloxacin has also been associated with the emergence of resistant bacterial strains (particularly Enterococci, pseudomonas and MRSA) (Hyatt and Schentag 2000; MacGowan et al. 2000; Zhou et al. 2000), and for gram-negative bacteria, this may occur when $AUC_{0-24h}/MIC <$ 100 (Thomas et al. 1998; Schentag 1999). Other studies have also shown that a high AUC_{0-24}/MIC can reduce the development of resistance with quinolone antibiotics (Ross et al. 2001; Tam et al. 2005; LaPlante et al. 2007).

The mutant prevention concentration (MPC) is defined as the drug concentration required to prevent emergence of all single step mutations in a population of at least 10^{10} bacterial cells (Zhao and Drlica 2001). Therefore, at drug concentrations above the MPC, at least a second step mutation is required for bacterial survival. Consequently, the MPC represents an important target for determining optimal dosing regimens that will minimize the selection of drug-resistant organisms (Dong et al. 1999). If drug levels are maintained at concentrations between the MIC and MPC for an organism, there is selective antibiotic pressure favouring the growth of single-step resistant mutants. This range of antibiotic concentrations is referred to as the mutant selection window (MSW) (Zhao and Drlica 2001) and has been defined for many of the fluoroquinolones and some β-lactams against various organisms (Firsov et al. 2003, 2006; Knudsen et al. 2003; Zinner et al. 2003; Croisier et al. 2004; Olofsson et al. 2006). The clinical relevance of the MSW remains unclear although future dosing regimes will likely focus on optimizing drug exposure to minimize the development of antibioitic resistance (Olofsson and Cars 2007).

Sub-optimal dosing of aminoglycosides may lead to adaptive resistance by virtue of a period of reduced drug uptake by the microorganism. Dosing to achieve improved C_{max}/MIC ratios appear to reduce this (Daikos et al. 1991; Xiong et al. 1997), although this is probably more a function of extended dosing intervals. In vitro data from Henderson-Begg et al. have also demonstrated that bacterial mutability can occur with sub-therapeutic aminoglycoside exposure (Henderson-Begg et al. 2006). Development of resistance has also been documented for carbapenems (Fink et al. 1994), and extended infusions may be more beneficial (Roberts et al. 2007b).

Existing dosing regimes for many antibiotics used in crtically ill patients will need re-evaulation in the context of onging investigation in this area. Many patients may be potentially under-dosed, with subsequent selection of resistant mutants. Higher doses, albeit within the limits of patient tolerability, must be considered in order to optimize patient response and prevent the development of further resistant infections.

8.7   Antibiotic Classes

Below, aminoglycosides, β-lactams, glycopepetides, fluoroquinolones and other various antibiotics used in critically ill patients with sepsis and septic shock are considered. General PK and PD characteristics have been tabulated for ease of reference for the reader (Table 8.1). A summary of the potential effects of the septic state on drug handling, clinical application and dosing implications for critically ill patients is also addressed (see Table 8.2).

Table 8.2 Changes in PK characteristics with sepsis and organ dysfunction, and implications for dosing

Antibiotic	Increase in Vd with sepsis	Decrease in C_{max} with fluid shifts	Clearance in sepsis without organ dysfunction	Effects of organ dysfunction	Possible dosing adjustments in severe sepsis	Therapeutic drug monitoring
Aminoglycosides	Yes (Nuytinck et al. 1988; Gosling et al. 1994; Buijk et al. 2002a)	Yes	↑ (Beckhouse et al. 1988; Bakker-Woudenberg and Roosendaal 1990; Triginer et al. 1990; Dager 1994)	↓ CL with renal dysfunction	↑ dose/↑ dosing frequency (with rapid CL)	Yes (Prins et al. 1993; Begg et al. 1995; Nicolau et al. 1995)
β-Lactams	Yes (Kieft et al. 1993; Joynt et al. 2001; Lipman et al. 2001)	Yes	↑	↓ CL with renal dysfunction (Barbhaiya et al. 1992; McKindley et al. 1996; Lipman et al. 2003)	↑ dosing frequency/infusion	No
Carbepenems	Yes (Mouton et al. 2000; Kitzes-Cohen et al. 2002; Novelli et al. 2005)	Yes	↑ (Mouton et al. 2000; Kitzes-Cohen et al. 2002; Novelli et al. 2005)	↓ CL with renal dysfunction (Gibson et al. 1985; Konishi et al. 1991; Leroy et al. 1992; Mouton et al. 2000)	↑ dosing frequency/infusion	No
Vancomycin	Yes	Yes	↑	↓ CL with renal dysfunction (Riley 1970; Matzke et al. 1984; Elting et al. 1998)	↑ dose (40 mg/kg/day IV)	Yes (ensure trough > 15mg/L)
Teicoplanin	Yes	Yes	↑	↓ CL with renal dysfunction	6 mg/kg IV 12-hourly × 3, then 6 mg/kg IV daily	Yes (Wilson 2000; Rybak 2006)

Tigecycline	Unlikely	Unlikely	Unlikely	↓ CL with cholelithiasis	100 mg LD, then 50 mg IV 12-hourly	No
Quinupristin/ dalfopristin	Yes	Yes	Unknown	Unknown	7.5 mg/kg IV 8-hourly	No
Daptomycin	Yes	Yes	↑	↓ CL with moderate renal dysfunction	4 mg/kg IV daily	No
Telithromycin	Unknown	No	↑	↓ CL with moderate renal dysfunction	800 mg PO daily	No
Clindamycin	No	Yes	Unknown	↓ CL with hepatic dysfunction	600 mg IV 8-hourly	No
Linezolid	Yes	Yes	↑(Adembri et al. 2008)	No dose adjustment required	600 mg IV 12-hourly	No
Ciprofloxacin	No	Yes	Not influenced	↓ CL with renal impairment and intra-abdominal pathology	↑ Frequency dosing (400 mg IV 8-hourly)	No
Levofloxacin	No	Yes	Unknown	↓ CL with renal dysfunction	↑ dose (500– 1000 mg IV daily)	No
Moxifloxacin	No	Yes	Not influenced		400 mg IV daily	No
Gatifloxacin	No	Yes	Unknown	↓ CL with renal dysfunction	400 mg IV daily	No
Azithromycin	Unlikely	Unlikely	Unlikely	No dose adjustment with hepatic impairment (Mazzei et al. 1993)	500 mg IV daily	No

CL clearance; PO per oral dose; IV intra-venous dose; LD loading dose

8.7.1 Aminoglycosides

Aminoglycosides (gentamicin, tobramycin and amikacin) have three important properties: (a) high, widely spaced doses cause less toxicity than smaller more frequent doses (Zhanel and Ariano 1992; Barza et al. 1996; Munckhof et al. 1996; Ali and Goetz 1997; Bailey et al. 1997; Olsen et al. 2004); (b) high doses produce better kill curves and clinical response (Moore et al. 1987) and (c) a significant PAE, limiting bacterial re-growth should drug concentrations fall below the MIC (Vogelman and Craig 1985, 1986; Moore et al. 1987; Vogelman et al. 1988; Roosendaal et al. 1989; Rodvold 2001; Olsen et al. 2004; Mouton and Vinks 2005). Single daily dosing for aminoglycoside antibiotics (extended interval dosing – EIAD) has been shown in prospective human clinical trials (Marik et al. 1991a,b; Van der Auwera et al. 1991; Prins et al. 1993; Olsen et al. 2004) and numerous meta-analyses (Barza et al. 1996; Munckhof et al. 1996; Ali and Goetz 1997; Bailey et al. 1997) to produce less toxicity and comparable if not superior clinical outcomes. This is also established in patients with organ dysfunction (Barclay et al. 1994; Hatala et al. 1997; Fisman and Kaye 2000).

In vitro studies have shown enhanced bacterial phagocytosis by leukocytes after exposure to aminoglycosides (post-antibiotic leukocyte enhancement – PALE) (McDonald et al. 1981). Neutropenia or a low leukocyte count, as shown in animal models (Kapusnik et al. 1988), may render aminoglycosides less effective (Klatersky 1986). However, specific dose modifications cannot be commended at this time.

Administration of high dose (7 mg/kg if normal renal function; amikacin requires 28 mg/kg) once-daily aminoglycosides is recommended. However, in our experience, where renal function is supra-normal and trough-level monitoring suggests that doses higher than 7 mg/kg are required, increasing the frequency to 18-hourly rather than an increased dose should be considered. The C_{max}/MIC ratio conferred by 7 mg/kg is generally at least 10, thereby maximizing bacterial killing (Kashuba et al. 1999; Rodvold 2001; Buijk et al. 2002a). Higher doses probably have no additional bactericidal effect. With renal impairment, dose reductions to 3–5 mg/kg 24-hourly may be required. Longer dosing intervals (36- or 48-hourly) may be necessary if this lower dose is inadequately excreted. Monitoring by trough levels should occur in this situation, although alternative agents can be considered. Variability in peak aminoglycoside plasma concentrations in critically ill patients (Zaske et al. 1980; Chelluri and Jastremski 1987; Mann et al. 1987a; Beckhouse et al. 1988; Dasta and Armstrong 1988; Fuhs et al. 1988; Chelluri et al. 1989; Reed et al. 1989; Townsend et al. 1989; Triginer et al. 1990; Dager 1994) may be due to an increased Vd (Table 8.2), and is correlated with illness severity (Marik 1993). This underscores the need for therapeutic drug monitoring.

Although in "normal" ward patients there are various methods for monitoring aminoglycoside dosing, including trough levels, published nomograms (Begg et al. 1995) and Bayesian computer software (Burton et al. 1985; Duffull et al. 1997; Kirkpatrick et al. 2003), their applicability in the critically ill is limited due to changes in Vd or the need for non-conventional dosing. Such situations require ensuring trough levels are <0.5 mg/L (preferably undetectable) prior to subsequent dosing. Some consideration to minimizing the duration of therapy is also important, as the total dose of aminoglycoside is strongly correlated with the risk of both ototoxicity and nephrotoxicity.

8.7.2   β-Lactam Antibiotics

The β-lactam group of antibiotics consists of penicillins, cephalosporins, carbapenems and monobactams. Carbapenems will be considered separately because of their different pharmacodynamic properties. With the time-dependent kill characteristics of β-lactams (Nuytinck et al. 1988), once the antibiotic concentration falls below the MIC, any remaining bacteria multiply almost immediately (Craig 1984; Schentag et al. 1984; Vogelman and Craig 1985, 1986; Vogelman et al. 1988; Leggett et al. 1989; Roosendaal et al. 1989; Bakker-Woudenberg and Roosendaal 1990; Mouton et al. 1997). In the absence of any PAE, the serum concentration of a β-lactam antibiotic should exceed the MIC for 90–100% of the dosing interval (Turnidge 1998b). Concentrations of β-lactam antibiotics should be maintained at 4–5 times the MIC during each dosing period (Vogelman and Craig 1985, 1986) as bacterial killing is maximal at these concentrations (Mouton and den Hollander 1994; Angus et al. 2000).

Unlike aminoglycosides, neutropenia may not reduce the antibacterial effect of β-lactams significantly, but relapse of infection when antibiotic therapy is ceased is documented (Roosendaal et al. 1986; Craig 2003). This supports the common practice of continuing β-lactam therapy until the patient's white cell count normalizes. Standard bolus administration (for example, of cephalosporins) produces unnecessary peak and trough concentrations below the MIC for much of the dosing interval (Young et al. 1997; Lipman et al. 1999a,b, 2001). It follows that an improved PD profile is obtained with either more frequent dosing (Turnidge 1998b; Lipman et al. 1999b) or continuous infusions (Mouton et al. 1997; Young et al. 1997; MacGowan and Bowker 1998; Turnidge 1998b; Georges et al. 1999; Lipman et al. 1999a,b; Tessier et al. 1999; Angus et al. 2000; Burgess et al. 2000; Jaruratanasirikul et al. 2002; Boselli et al. 2003; Tam et al. 2003).

Sepsis without organ dysfunction can lead to increased β-lactam clearance and low plasma concentrations (Bakker-Woudenberg and Roosendaal 1990; Young et al. 1997; MacGowan and Bowker 1998; Gomez et al. 1999; Lipman et al. 1999a,b, 2001; Angus et al. 2000; Hanes et al. 2000). In two of these studies, the clearance of cefepime and more recently cefpirome, were linearly correlated with creatinine clearance (Lipman et al. 1999b, 2001). PK–PD modeling found that the T > MIC could be predicted by creatinine clearance, and that plasma concentrations of these antibiotics were low when using a standard dosing regimen (Lipman et al. 1999b, 2001). Dosing adjustment according to increased renal function is an important PK consideration to ensure optimal therapy, and may require increased dosing, or preferably increased frequency of dosing to ensure T > MIC is maximized.

Furthermore, an increased Vd in the critically ill (Gomez et al. 1999; Hanes et al. 2000) demands dosage adjustment (Table 8.2). Joukhadar et al. (2001) showed that an increased Vd in patients with septic shock results in unbound piperacillin concentrations that can be 5–10 times lower in the extracellular fluid of subcutaneous tissue compared with serum levels after a piperacillin bolus dose.

Administration by continuous infusion optimizes the PD profile of β-lactams (Mouton and den Hollander 1994; Fry 1996; Lipman et al. 1996; Mouton et al. 1997; Turnidge 1998b). Numerous studies have been performed comparing administration by continuous infusion versus bolus dosing (Mouton et al. 1997; Angus et al. 2000; Hanes et al. 2000; McNabb et al. 2001; Nicolau et al. 2001; Georges et al. 2005; Lorente et al. 2005a; Roberts et al. 2007a,b). These have largely shown comparable therapeutic efficacy, although Roberts et al. in their prospective randomized controlled trial found clinical and bacteriologic superiority when administering ceftriaxone 2-g as a continuous intravenous infusion compared to a once-daily bolus dose in patients receiving four or more days of treatment (Roberts et al. 2007a). Continuous infusion has also been reported to result in a reduction in total daily dose; shorter duration of treatment (MacGowan and Bowker 1998); decreased nursing time for administration; possible reduction in formation of resistant bacteria (Young et al. 1997; Klepser et al. 1998) and lower expenditure on patient therapy(Kollef et al. 1999; Krueger et al. 2002).

Recently, Lodise and colleagues performed a retrospective cohort study in 194 critically ill patients with *Pseudomonas aeruginosa* infections, receiving piperacillin-tazobactam by intermittent infusion (over 30 min) or extended infusion (over 3 h) (Lodise et al. 2007). In patients with an APACHE II score greater than 17 ($n = 79$), use of an extended infusion had a lower 14-day mortality rate (12.2% vs. 31.6%; $p = 0.04$) (Lodise et al. 2007). It is likely that the clinical advantage for infusion will be most notable in critically ill patients being treated for gram-negative infections. The benefit of continous- or extended infusions in this setting probably relates to the lack of a significant PAE of β-lactams (except carbapenems) against these organisms.

8.7.3 Carbapenems

Carbapenems (meropenem, imipenem and panipenem) are a separate class of β-lactam antibiotics. In similarity with other β-lactams, they demonstrate time-dependent killing (Table 8.1) and have minimal side effects (Mouton et al. 2000). Increased seizure activity has been noted with imipenem and is a potential adverse effect for all carbapenems, particularly in infants, the elderly and those with renal impairment (Barrons et al. 1992; Day et al. 1995; Norrby et al. 1995; Laethem et al. 2003). In vitro models have shown that carbapenems require less T > MIC for bacteriostatic activity (20%) and bactericidal activity (40%) (Drusano 2003) as compared with other β-lactams. This is most likely secondary to the carbapenem PAE (Bustamante et al. 1984).

Administration by continuous infusion to maximize T > MIC remains a topical issue for carbapenems particularly as this seems less important compared to other β-lactams. Some preliminary data suggest clinical superiority of administration by continuous infusion in critically ill patients (Lorente et al. 2005b) with avoidance of concentration-related toxicity (Craig 1998; Drusano 2003) and pharmacoeconomic advantages from reduced total daily dose (Kotapati et al. 2004). Recently, Lorente et al. performed a retrospective cohort study in 89 patietns with gram-negative bacilli ventilator-associated pneumonia treated with meropenem administered by bolus or continuous infusion (Lorente et al. 2006). This paper described superior clinical cure rates in the continuous infusion group compared with the bolus group (90.5% vs. 59.6%; $p < 0.001$) (Lorente et al. 2006). The principal disadvantage is drug stability for 24-h infusions. Meropenem may only be stable for a maximum of 8 h requiring a new infusion to be made when a bolus would normally be administered (Thalhammer et al. 1999; Krueger et al. 2005). Generally a designated intravenous line to avoid drug incompatibility problems is required. Further prospective research to determine the clinical efficacy of administering carbapenems as a continuous or extended infusion is required.

8.7.4 Glycopeptides

The specific interpretation of the PD properties of glycopeptides is not fully understood. Vancomycin will be preferentially discussed as representative of the glycopeptides due to its more prevalent usage. Vancomycin is well known to induce PAE and has PD properties in common with both aminoglycosides and β-lactams. Some data suggest that the bactericidal activity of vancomycin is time dependent (Saunders 1994; Larsson et al. 1996; Lowdin et al. 1998). Similar results have been obtained for teicoplanin in a rabbit endocarditis model (Chambers and Kennedy 1990). However, an in vitro study (Duffull et al. 1994) found no difference in rates of killing of $S.$ $aureus$ by vancomycin when given as continuous infusion or bolus dose suggesting that T > MIC is not necessary for optimal bacterial killing. $C_{max}/$MIC was found to predict efficacy in a non-neutropenic mouse peritonitis model for $S.$ $pneumoniae$ and $S.$ $aureus$ suggesting that glycopeptides might show concentration-dependent killing against some organisms (Knudsen et al. 2000). Whether this PD effect is primarily due to the presence of neutrophils in this model is unknown.

Other studies have proposed that $AUC_{0-24}/$MIC is the most important PK–PD parameter correlating with efficacy for vancomycin (Craig 2003; Rybak 2006). As such, the optimal dosing regimen for administration of vancomycin remains unknown (Duffull et al. 1994; Saunders 1994; James et al. 1996; Wysocki et al. 2001; Rello et al. 2005). The data is confused, as despite adequate vancomycin trough concentrations being maintained by dosing 6-, 8- or 12-hourly or by continuous infusion, there is a lack of definitive evidence of PD efficacy and no evidence linking concentrations to either outcome or toxicity (Saunders 1994; MacGowan 1998). Wysocki et al.

(2001) find no significant difference in clinical efficacy between continuous infusions and bolus dosing, but Rello et al. (2005) described the clinical superiority of continuous vancomycin infusions in a subset of patients treated for ventilator-associated pneumonia caused by methicillin-resistant *Staphylococcus aureus* (MRSA). Thus, while the economic advantages of reduced dosage of vancomycin by continuous infusion have been described (Wysocki et al. 2001), the clinical relevance of this remains unclear. However, dosing strategies to improve AUC_{0-24}/MIC in critically ill patients with neutropaenia may be prudent, as research suggests this is the most important PD parameter in animal neutropenic models (Rybak 2006).

To optimize dosing of vancomycin in critically ill patients with sepsis, maintenance of trough levels of at least 15–20 mg/L are required (MacGowan 1998). In our experience, higher doses than those conventionally recommended (similar to paediatric doses of 40 mg/kg/day) may be needed to optimize plasma concentrations (Gous et al. 1995). For teicoplanin, when there is no renal impairment, dosing at 6 mg/kg 12-hourly for three doses, followed by 6 mg/kg 24-hourly thereafter, is recommended. Therapeutic drug monitoring is indicated only when high doses (12 mg/kg/day) are used or to avoid toxicity. Current practice suggests that teicoplanin concentrations be maintained above 10 mg/L (15–20 mg/L for endocarditis) (Rybak 2006).

Vancomycin poorly penetrates into solid organs, particularly the lung (Cruciani et al. 1996; Bodi et al. 2001). Thus, if the source of sepsis is thought to be in the lung, the co-prescription of rifampicin as dual therapy has been advocated (Burnie et al. 2000; Bodi et al. 2001). Therapy with rifampicin is frequently avoided due to its potential for drug interactions through CYP3A4 inuduction. Use as a single agent is not recommended because of its propensity to cause bacterial resistance (Lipman 2005). Alternatively, high dose vancomycin (aiming for trough concentrations ≥20 mg/L) has been suggested (Lipman 2005) for sepsis originating in solid organs. Other antibacterial agents provide better penetration of the epithelial lining fluid of the lung and thus therapy with either fusidic acid (Turnidge 1999), linezolid (Conte et al. 2002), tigecycline (Peterson 2005) or televancin (Reyes et al. 2005) may be preferred. Teicoplanin does not provide any specific clinical advantages and newer drugs will likely take its place as a vancomycin subsititute.

8.7.5 Fluoroquinolones

Fluoroquinolone antibiotics include ciprofloxacin, moxifloxacin, levofloxacin and gatifloxacin. These are a relatively new class of antibiotics, and other than for ciprofloxacin, there is little data to guide dosing in critically ill patients. As such, ciprofloxacin will be discussed in preference where information is not available.

Although achieving a C_{max}/MIC ratio of 10 for ciprofloxacin is the critical variable in predicting bacterial eradication (Preston et al. 1998), Forrest et al. (1993) concluded that achieving an AUC_{0-24hr}/MIC > 125 is associated with a successful clinical outcome in critically ill patients with gram-negative infections. For gram-positive organisms, an AUC_{0-24hr}/MIC of only 30 is required (Nix et al. 1992; Forrest et al. 1993; Piddock and Dalhoff 1993; Goss et al. 1994), although fluoroquinolones should not be used as single agent treatment of gram-positive infections. The dose recommended to achieve these PD parameters for ciprofloxacin is 400 mg IV 8-hourly in adults and this need not be changed during sepsis unless renal dysfunction occurs (Lipman et al. 1998; Gous et al. 2005). However, pharmacodynamic analysis has shown that this maximum dose has a 55% probability of achieving the AUC target of 125 (Sun et al. 2005) and as such larger doses or different dosing regimens may be recommended in the future. There is growing evidence for increased dosing of levofloxacin in critically ill patients with sepsis (1,000 mg daily) (Viale and Pea 2003; Graninger and Zeitlinger 2004), and with more safety and efficacy data, further increases in recommended doses may occur for other fluoroquinolone antibiotics as well.

All fluoroquinolone antibiotics demonstrate good tissue penetration (Gous et al. 2005). Ciprofloxacin is hepatically metabolized, although dose adjustment is recommended by the manufacturers' product information (MIMS Australia 2005b) in renal dysfunction to prevent accumulation of drug and metabolites (Hoffken et al. 1985). However, Jones has shown impaired ciprofloxacin clearance with renal impairment only when the patient had concomitant bowel or liver pathology (Jones 1997).

As referenced in previous sections of this chapter, under-dosing of fluoroquinolones may be implicated in selecting resistant sub-populations of infecting organsims. Although dosing to achieve specific pharmacodynamic end points has been associated with improved outcomes (Forrest et al. 1993), higher doses or alternative dosing regimens may be needed to minimize the development of resistance. Achieving a high $AUC_{0-24hrs}$/MPC has been shown to predict the prevention of resistant mutants (Olofsson et al. 2006), and may become the aim of dosing strategies in the future.

8.7.6 Tigecycline

Tigecycline is a member of the glycylcyclines which are novel tetracyclines with gram-positive and gram-negative activity. Tigecycline has shown rapid and extensive penetration into body tissues, and was shown to have 74% penetration into inflammatory fluid (Meagher et al. 2005a). Tigecycline displays time-dependent killing against *Streptoccus pneumoniae, Haemophilus influenzae* and *Neisseria gonorrhea* (Petersen et al. 1999) but AUC_{0-24}/MIC is more likely to be correlated with efficacy (Meagher et al. 2005a,b), due to the agent's long half-life and prolonged PAE. More research into the pharmacodynamic principles of tigecycline is needed.

Tigecycline should be reserved for infections caused by multi-resistant organisms. While a higher (100 mg loading dose then 50 mg 12-hourly) and lower dosing regimen (50 mg loading dose then 25 mg 12-hourly) has been previously trialled (Postier et al. 2004), the superior clinical and bacteriologic success of the higher dosing regimen suggests that it may be more suitable for critically ill patients with sepsis.

8.7.7   Telithromycin

Telithromycin is the first ketolide marketed and has properties very similar to macrolide antibiotics. Telithromycin has been shown to have good extracellular penetration with therapeutic levels in respiratory tissues (Muller-Serieys et al. 2004), sites of inflammation (blister fluids 38% above plasma (Namour et al. 2002)) and in neutrophils (Kasbekar and Acharya 2005). However, poor penetration in muscle and adipose tissue (Gattringer et al. 2004) has been reported. Telithromycin also exhibits long post-antibiotic effects and post-antibiotic sub-MIC effects enabling once-daily dosing (Odenholt et al. 2001; Jacobs et al. 2003).

No evidence exists to support altered dosing in patients with "third spacing", and current evidence suggests that no dose adjustments are required in patients based on weight (Shi et al. 2004). In moderate to severe renal impairment (CrCL 30 ml/min), doses should be halved (from 800 mg 24-hourly to 400 mg 24-hourly) (Shi et al. 2004). No dose adjustment is required in hepatic disease (Kasbekar and Acharya 2005). Telithromycin is a potent inhibitor of the metabolic enzyme CYP3A4 and should be used with caution with midazolam and triazolam (potential to prolong Q-Tc), HMG-CoA reductase inhibitors or "statins" (risk of myopathy), digoxin, metoprolol and theophylline (elevated drug levels). Phenytoin and other enzyme inducers may reduce telithromycin levels. Telithromycin is available only in oral dosage form and is recommended at 800 mg daily for 7–10 days for community-acquired pneumonia.

8.7.8   Azithromycin

Azithromycin is a macrolide derivative more appropriately referred to as an "azalide" antibiotic, and is most commonly employed in the treatment of atypical respiratory pathogens in patients presenting with severe community-acquired pneumonia. Its structure in comparison with macrolides results in greater tissue penetration and longer plasma half-life, increased activity against gram-negative organisms and decreased activity against some gram-positive organisms (Piscitelli et al. 1992). Mean tissue concentrations are 10–100-fold greater than plasma concentrations (Foulds et al. 1990). Azithromycin is also actively taken up by white blood cells that carry the antibiotic to the site of infection (Amsden 1996).

AUC_{24}/MIC appears to be the PD parameter most closely associated with clinical efficacy, although concentrations at the site of infection rather than in plasma are more likely to correlate with antimicrobial effects (Firsov et al. 2002). Recent work has suggested that AUC_{24}/MIC values ≥ 25 are needed to achieve and maintain bactericidal activity against *S. pneumoniae* (Sevillano et al. 2006). Given the extensive tissue distribution of azithromycin, changes in Vd are unlikely to occur with severe sepsis, although there is no data currently available on the PK changes of this agent in the critically ill. The recommended dose is 500 mg daily for 3–5 days in the treatment of suspected atypical pneumonia.

8.7.9   Daptomycin

Daptomycin is a novel lipopolypetide antimicrobial agent with good activity against most gram-positive pathogens. Although it was discovered 20 years ago, it has been marketed only recently with limited clinical studies to provide data on toxicity. Dosing should be adjusted in renal impairment. Early trials correlated muscle weakness, myalgia and marked increases in creatinine phosphokinase (CPK) with 12-hourly dosing (Tally et al. 1999), leading to the present recommendation of 4 mg/kg/24 h by intravenous daily bolus.

C_{max}/MIC is the PD parameter associated with clinical efficacy (Safdar et al. 2004). Daptomycin has a prolonged PAE of 2–6 h in MSSA and MRSA (Pankuch et al. 2003) and 1–2.5 h in *S. pneumoniae* (Safdar et al. 2004). Distribution is likely to be limited to the extracellular fluid spaces and third spacing may result in reduced C_{max}. It distributes rapidly into inflammatory fluid but does not reach the plasma concentrations, probably due to differences in the protein content of this fluid (Wise et al. 2002). If patients develop moderate to severe renal impairment (CrCl < 30 ml/min), then the frequency should be extended to 48-hourly dosing (Schriever et al. 2005). The effect of hypoalbuminaemia in hepatic impairment on unbound daptomycin concentration remains unknown, but patients should be monitored for changes in CPK if this occurs.

It has been suggested that daptomycin requires the presence of free calcium ions in a growth medium for activity against gram-positive organisms (Andrew et al. 1987). The effect this may have in humans with low serum calcium concentrations is unknown. In the acutely septic presents with low serum calcium levels, consideration should be given to correcting the serum calcium concentration and closely monitoring the clinical response. Daptomycin should be reserved for serious infections caused by MRSA, VRE and MRSE that do not respond to vancomycin.

8.7.10   Quinupristin/Dalfopristin

Quinupristin/dalfopristin (Q/D) is a combination of two injectable streptogrammins with demonstrated efficacy against multi-resistant gram-positive organisms. In vitro studies have shown significant CYP3A4 inhibition by Q/D, and care should be exercised when administering other drugs that are also inhibitors, substrates for, or inducers of this enzyme system (MIMS Australia 2005a). Q/D is thought to have concentration-dependent efficacy with 99.9% killing of isolates of vancomycin-resistant *Enterococcus faecium* (VREF) in vitro best correlated a high ratio of Q/D concentration to minimum bactericidal concentration (MBC) (Aeschlimann and Rybak 1998). Some authors have suggested that AUC_{0-24}/MIC is the primary parameter correlated with efficacy (Craig 2001). Hepatic dysfunction may result in altered metabolism of Q/D or may cause unpredictable effects from other CYP3A4 metabolized drugs from unknown inhibition.

Little information exists to guide dosing of quinupristin/dalfopristin in critically ill patients with sepsis. If penetration to the infection site is considered impaired, then co-administration with another antibiotic (e.g. linezolid or a glycopeptide) is recommended (De Gaudio and Di Filippo 2003). Q/D is recommended to be dosed at 7.5 mg/kg intravenous administration 8-hourly for VREF and 7.5 mg/kg intravenous administration 12-hourly for complicated skin and skin structure infections with *Staphylococcus aureus* (methicillin-susceptible) (MIMS Australia 2005a).

8.7.11   Lincosamides

The lincosamide antibiotics include clindamycin and lincomycin. Clindamycin is widely distributed throughout the body and achieves therapeutic concentrations in most body compartments (Fass and Saslaw 1972; Nagar et al. 1989; Mueller et al. 1999). It is extensively hepatically metabolized and renally excreted with its clearance reduced in hepatic dysfunction (Avant et al. 1975). Lincomycin has similar properties to clindamycin although distribution into tissues may not be as wide (Gwilt and Smith 1986). While lincomycin is also extensively hepatically metabolized (Bellamy et al. 1967), its clearance is reduced in both severe renal and hepatic impairment (Bellamy et al. 1967).

T > MIC has been determined to be the pharmacodynamic factor correlated with efficacy. Free drug levels of lincosamides should exceed the MIC of the infective pathogen for at least 40–50% of the dosing interval (Craig 2001). Lincosamides are indicated for suspected/confirmed anaerobic infections in critically ill patients with sepsis due to their extensive distribution characteristics. Standard doses should be used for clindamycin (1,200–2,700 mg in three or four divided doses) unless significant hepatic impairment is present. Lincomycin dosing (600–2,400 mg 8-hourly dependent on the severity of infection) should be reduced in the presence of either significant renal or hepatic impairment.

8.7.12   Linezolid

Linezolid is the first of a new class of antimicrobials called the oxazolinediones. It widely distributes into tissues including inflammatory fluids, extracellular lining fluid and CSF (MacGowan 2003; Boselli et al. 2005). Linezolid is mostly metabolized and then renally cleared although no dose adjustment is recommended in renal dysfunction (Brier et al. 2003) or hepatic dysfunction (MacGowan 2003).

In animal models, T > MIC was the major predictor of efficacy with *S. pneumoniae* in a murine thigh infection model (Andes et al. 1998) and a rat pneumonia model(Gentry-Nielsen et al. 2002). In both models T > MIC of 40–45% was the best predictor of outcome. Subsequent animal models using *S. pneumoniae*, *S. aureus* and pneumococci have predicted that an AUC_{0-24}/MIC ratio of 50–80 correlate well with efficacy (Andes et al. 2002). A 600-mg 12-hourly dose should achieve this ratio in humans against susceptible organisms with MICs up to 2–4 mg/L. There is some information to suggest that maximal *S. aureus* killing may occur with T > MIC for 100% of the dosing interval (Craig 2003).

Linezolid can effect warfarin activity resulting in a decrease in the mean international normalized ratio (INR) (Azie et al. 2000). As such warfarin dosing should be carefully monitored. Linezolid is also a reversible non-selective inhibitor of monoamine oxidase (MAO) (MacGowan 2003), and can have interactions with other inhibitors resulting in an uncontrolled vasopressor response.

In the majority of patients, linezolid is safe and well tolerated for up to 28 days at 600 mg twice daily (French 2003). Evidence exists that therapy longer than 14 days can rarely cause reversible myelosuppression (Gerson et al. 2002), although a causal relationship has not been established. As such patients prescribed linezolid should have blood counts ordered weekly if two or more weeks of treatment is indicated (French 2003).

8.8   PK/PD Modelling

As outlined in the previous sections of this chapter, severe sepsis can result in a number of changes in PK parameters for different antibiotics. As such, Vd and clearance for these agents can be notably different in this patient population compared with healthy volunteers. In addition, inter-individual variation can be substantial, and individualization of the dosing regimen may be necessary to achieve optimal results. Determining creatinine clearance (as a key marker of drug elimination) and mathematical modelling of drug distribution will allow tailoring of dosing regimens to individual patients.

The application of pharmacokinetic/pharmacodynamic modelling in guiding the individualization of antibiotic doses in critically ill patients with nosocomial gram-negative infections has been investigated (Mohr et al. 2004). In their study, Mohr et al. demonstrated the applicability of mathematical modelling to achieve optimal PD profiles in individual patients, and subsequent clinical and microbiological improvement (Mohr et al. 2004). Similarly, creatinine clearance has recently been demonstrated to be a good marker of cefpirome clearance and could potentially be used to individualize cefpirome therapy (Roos et al. 2007). Recent work by Dailly et al. has recommended the use of a simple formula for individualizing ceftazidime dosage administered by continuous infusion in patients with haematological malignancies (Dailly et al. 2006). This work serves to underscore the importance of considering PD and PK parameters in dosing of antibiotics in critically ill patients and further work is needed to allow early identification of high risk patients.

8.9 Conclusion

Current antibiotic regimens have mostly been derived from trials with patients who are not critically ill. Optimizing antibiotic regimens in patients with sepsis requires an understanding of the pathophysiological changes that affect antibiotic dosing in severe sepsis and the different kill characteristics of the various antibiotic classes.

Certain antibiotics may have a high Vd, and hence lead to a low C_{max} during sepsis. It follows that under-dosing may occur if a high peak is needed (e.g. aminoglycosides).

The Vd of antibiotics that distribute primarily into extravascular water, namely aminoglycosides, vancomycin and, to a lesser extent, β-lactams, changes with clinical illness severity. Dosing may need to be altered during the course of illness irrespective of renal or hepatic function, something not commonly described for non-critically ill patients.

In many critically ill patients, despite a normal serum creatinine, supra-normal creatinine clearance, and as a consequence more rapid drug elimination can be demonstrated. High drug clearances lead to sub-therapeutic levels and increase the likelihood of treatment failure and the development of resistant microorganisms. In relation to the aminoglycosides, this means that not only are large doses required to be administered, but these antibiotics may also need dosing more frequently. Similarly, β-lactams and fluroquinolones should, in such patients, be dosed more frequently than suggested in non-sepsis patients.

Treatment of sepsis remains a significant challenge given persistently high mortality and morbidity rates. Data suggest that effective antibiotic therapy remains the most important intervention available to the clinician. In treating sepsis, the clinician must be cognizant of the various pathophysiological and subsequent PK–PD changes that can occur, and how these may influence drug concentration, and hence outcome.

References

Adembri C, Fallani S, Cassetta MI, et al. (2008) Linezolid pharmacokinetic/pharmacodynamic profile in critically ill septic patients: intermittent versus continuous infusion. Int J Antimicrob Agents 31: 122–129.

Aeschlimann JR and Rybak MJ (1998) Pharmacodynamic analysis of the activity of quinupristin-dalfopristin against vancomycin-resistant Enterococcus faecium with differing MBCs via time-kill-curve and postantibiotic effect methods. Antimicrob Agents Chemother 42: 2188–2192.

Ali MZ and Goetz MB (1997) A meta-analysis of the relative efficacy and toxicity of single daily dosing versus multiple daily dosing of aminoglycosides. Clin Infect Dis 24: 796–809.

Amsden GW (1996) Erythromycin, clarithromycin, and azithromycin: are the differences real? Clin Ther 18: 56–72; discussion 55.

Andes D, van Ogtrop ML, and Craig W (1998) Pharmacodynamic activity of a new oxazolidinone linezolid in an animal infection model. 38th Interscience Conference on Antimicrobial Agents and Chemotherapy, American Society for Microbiology, San Diego, CA.

Andes D, van Ogtrop ML, Peng J, et al. (2002) In vivo pharmacodynamics of a new oxazolidinone (linezolid). Antimicrob Agents Chemother 46: 3484–3489.

Andrew JH, Wale MC, Wale LJ, et al. (1987) The effect of cultural conditions on the activity of LY146032 against staphylococci and streptococci. J Antimicrob Chemother 20: 213–221.

Angus BJ, Smith MD, Suputtamongkol Y, et al. (2000) Pharmacokinetic-pharmacodynamic evaluation of ceftazidime continuous infusion vs intermittent bolus injection in septicaemic melioidosis. Br J Clin Pharmacol 50: 184–191.

Athamna A, Athamna M, Medlej B, et al. (2004) In vitro post-antibiotic effect of fluoroquinolones, macrolides, beta-lactams, tetracyclines, vancomycin, clindamycin, linezolid, chloramphenicol, quinupristin/dalfopristin and rifampicin on Bacillus anthracis. J Antimicrob Chemother 53: 609–615.

Avant GR, Schenker S, and Alford RH (1975) The effect of cirrhosis on the disposition and elimination of clindamycin. Am J Dig Dis 20: 223–230.

Azie NE, Stalker DJ, Jungbluth GL, et al. (2000) Effect of linezolid on CYP2C9 using racemic warfarin as a probe. Abstract PI-81. Clin Pharmacol Ther 69: 21.

Bailey TC, Little JR, Littenberg B, et al. (1997) A meta-analysis of extended-interval dosing versus multiple daily dosing of aminoglycosides. Clin Infect Dis 24: 786–795.

Bakker-Woudenberg IA and Roosendaal R (1990) Impact of dosage schedule of antibiotics on the treatment of serious infections. Intensive Care Med 16: S229–S234.

Barbhaiya RH, Forgue ST, Gleason CR, et al. (1992) Pharmacokinetics of cefepime after single and multiple intravenous administrations in healthy subjects. Antimicrob Agents Chemother 36: 552–557.

Barbot A, Venisse N, Rayeh F, et al. (2003) Pharmacokinetics and pharmacodynamics of sequential intravenous and subcutaneous teicoplanin in critically ill patients without vasopressors. Intensive Care Med 29: 1528–1534.

Barclay ML, Begg EJ, and Hickling KG (1994) What is the evidence for once-daily aminoglycoside therapy? Clin Pharmacokinet 27: 32–48.

Barrons RW, Murray KM, and Richey RM (1992) Populations at risk for penicillin-induced seizures. Ann Pharmacother 26: 26–29.

Bartlett JG, Dowell SF, Mandell LA, et al. (2000) Practice guidelines for the management of community-acquired pneumonia in adults. Infectious Diseases Society of America. Clin Infect Dis 31: 347–382.

Barza M, Ioannidis JP, Cappelleri JC, et al. (1996) Single or multiple daily doses of aminoglycosides: a meta-analysis. BMJ 312: 338–345.

Beckhouse MJ, Whyte IM, Byth PL, et al. (1988) Altered aminoglycoside pharmacokinetics in the critically ill. Anaesth Intensive Care 16: 418–422.

Begg EJ, Barclay ML, and Duffull SB (1995) A suggested approach to once-daily aminoglycoside dosing. Br J Clin Pharmacol 39: 605–609.

Bellamy HMJ, Bates BB, and Reinarz JA (1967) Lincomycin metabolism in patients with hepatic insufficiency: effect of liver disease on lincomycin serum concentrations. Antimicrob Agents Chemother 7: 36.

Bennett WM, Aronoff GR, Golper TA, et al. (1994). Drug Prescribing in Renal Failure. American College of Physicians, Philadelphia.

Bernard E, Bensoussan M, Bensoussan F, et al. (1994) Pharmacokinetics and suction blister fluid penetration of a semisynthetic injectable streptogrammin. Eur J Clin Microbiol Infect Dis 13: 768–771.

Bodi M, Ardanuy C, Olona M, et al. (2001) Therapy of ventilator-associated pneumonia: the Tarragona strategy. Clin Microbiol Infect 7: 32–33.

Bone RC, Balk RA, Cerra FB, et al. (1992) Definitions for sepsis and organ failure and guidelines for the use of innovative therapies in sepsis. The ACCP/SCCM Consensus Conference Committee. American College of Chest Physicians/Society of Critical Care Medicine. Chest 101: 1644–1655.

Boselli E, Breilh D, Duflo F, et al. (2003) Steady-state plasma and intrapulmonary concentrations of cefepime administered in continuous infusion in critically ill patients with severe nosocomial pneumonia. Crit Care Med 31: 2102–2106.

Boselli E, Breilh D, Rimmele T, et al. (2005) Pharmacokinetics and intrapulmonary concentrations of linezolid administered to critically ill patients with ventilator-associated pneumonia. Crit Care Med 33: 1529–1533.

Boucher BA, Kuhl DA, and Hickerson WL (1992) Pharmacokinetics of systemically administered antibiotics in patients with thermal injury. Clin Infect Dis 14: 458–463.

Bouvier d'Yvoire MJY and Maire PH (1996) Dosage regimens of antibacterials: implications of a pharmacokinetic/pharmacodynamic model. Clin Drug Investig 11: 229–239.

Brater DC, Bawdon RE, Anderson SA, et al. (1986) Vancomycin elimination in patients with burn injury. Clin Pharmacol Ther 39: 631–634.

Brier ME, Stalker DJ, Aronoff GR, et al. (2003) Pharmacokinetics of linezolid in subjects with renal dysfunction. Antimicrob Agents Chemother 47: 2775–2780.

Brittain DC, Scully BE, McElrath MJ, et al. (1985) The pharmacology of orally administered ciprofloxacin. Drugs Exp Clin Res 11: 339–341.

Brogden RN and Peters DH (1994) Teicoplanin. A reappraisal of its antimicrobial activity, pharmacokinetic properties and therapeutic efficacy. Drugs 47: 823–854.

Bugge JF (2001) Pharmacokinetics and drug dosing adjustments during continuous venovenous hemofiltration or hemodiafiltration in critically ill patients. Acta Anaesthesiol Scand 45: 929–934.

Buijk SE, Mouton JW, Gyssens IC, et al. (2002a) Experience with a once-daily dosing program of aminoglycosides in critically ill patients. Intensive Care Med 28: 936–942.

Buijk SL, Gyssens IC, Mouton JW, et al. (2002b) Pharmacokinetics of ceftazidime in serum and peritoneal exudate during continuous versus intermittent administration to patients with severe intra-abdominal infections. J Antimicrob Chemother 49: 121–128.

Burgess DS, Hastings RW, and Hardin TC (2000) Pharmacokinetics and pharmacodynamics of cefepime administered by intermittent and continuous infusion. Clin Ther 22: 66–75.

Burnie J, Matthews R, Jiman-Fatami A, et al. (2000) Analysis of 42 cases of septicemia caused by an epidemic strain of methicillin-resistant Staphylococcus aureus: evidence of resistance to vancomycin. Clin Infect Dis 31: 684–689.

Burton ME, Brater DC, Chen PS, et al. (1985) A Bayesian feedback method of aminoglycoside dosing. Clin Pharmacol Ther 37: 349–357.

Bustamante CI, Drusano GL, Tatem BA, et al. (1984) Postantibiotic effect of imipenem on Pseudomonas aeruginosa. Antimicrob Agents Chemother 26: 678–682.

Calandra T and Cohen J (2005) The international sepsis forum consensus conference on definitions of infection in the intensive care unit. Crit Care Med 33: 1538–1548.

Chambers HE and Sande MA (1996) Goodman and Gillman's The Pharmacological Basis of Therapeutics. McGraw Hill, New York.

Chambers HF and Kennedy S (1990) Effects of dosage, peak and trough concentrations in serum, protein binding, and bacterial rate on efficacy of teicoplanin in a rabbit model of endocarditis. Antimicrob Agents Chemother 47: 2018–2021.

Chant C and Rybak MJ (1995) Quinupristin/dalfopristin (RP 59500): a new streptogrammin antibiotic. Ann Pharmacother 29: 1022–1027.

Chelluri L and Jastremski MS (1987) Inadequacy of standard aminoglycoside loading doses in acutely ill patients. Crit Care Med 15: 1143–1145.

Chelluri L, Warren J, and Jastremski MS (1989) Pharmacokinetics of a 3 mg/kg body weight loading dose of gentamicin or tobramycin in critically ill patients. Chest 95: 1295–1297.

Chien SC, Chow AT, Natarajan J, et al. (1997) Absence of age and gender effects on the pharmacokinetics of a single 500-milligram oral dose of levofloxacin in healthy subjects. Antimicrob Agents Chemother 41: 1562–1565.

Chien SC, Wong FA, Fowler CL, et al. (1998) Double-blind evaluation of the safety and pharmacokinetics of multiple oral once-daily 750-milligram and 1-gram doses of levofloxacin in healthy volunteers. Antimicrob Agents Chemother 42: 885–888.

Chiu LM, Menhinick AM, Johnson PW, et al. (2002) Pharmacokinetics of intravenous azithromycin and ceftriaxone when administered alone and concurrently to healthy volunteers. J Antimicrob Chemother 50: 1075–1079.

Cockroft DW and Gault MH (1976) Prediction of creatinine clearance from serum creatinine. Nephron 16: 31–41.

Conte JE, Golden JA, Kipps J, et al. (2002) Intrapulmonary pharmacokinetics of linezolid. Antimicrob Agents Chemother 26: 1475–1480.

Craig W (1984) Pharmacokinetic and experimental data on beta-lactam antibiotics in the treatment of patients. Eur J Clin Microbiol Infect Dis 3: 575–578.

Craig WA (1993) Post-antibiotic effects in experimental infection models: relationship to in-vitro phenomena and to treatment of infections in man. J Antimicrob Chemother 31 Suppl D: 149–158.

Craig WA (1998) Pharmacokinetic/pharmacodynamic parameters: rationale for antibacterial dosing of mice and men. Clin Infect Dis 26: 1–10; quiz 11–12.

Craig WA (2001) Does the dose matter? Clin Infect Dis 33 Suppl 3: S233–S237.

Craig WA (2003) Basic pharmacodynamics of antibacterials with clinical applications to the use of b-lactams, glycopeptides, and linezolid. Infect Dis Clin North Am 17: 479–501.

Craig WA and Ebert SC (1991) Killing and regrowth of bacteria in vitro: a review. Scand J Infect Dis 74: 63–70.

Croisier D, Etienne M, Bergoin E, et al. (2004) Mutant selection window in levofloxacin and moxifloxacin treatments of experimental pneumococcal pneumonia in a rabbit model of human therapy. Antimicrob Agents Chemother 48: 1699–1707.

Cruciani M, Gatti G, Lazzarini L, et al. (1996) Penetration of vancomycin into human lung tissue. J Antimicrob Chemother 38: 865–869.

Cunha BA (1995a) Vancomycin. Med Clin North Am 79: 817–831.

Cunha BA (1995b) Antibiotic treatment of sepsis. Med Clin North Am 79: 551–558.

Dager WE (1994) Aminoglycoside pharmacokinetics: volume of distribution in specific adult patient subgroups. Ann Pharmacother 28: 944–951.

Daikos GL, Lolans VT, and Jackson GG (1991) First-exposure adaptive resistance to aminoglycoside antibiotics in vivo with meaning for optimal clinical use. Antimicrob Agents Chemother 35: 117–123.

Dailly E, Brun A, Kergueris MF, et al. (2006) A simple formula for individualising ceftazidime dosage administered by continuous infusion in patients with haematological malignancies. Int J Antimicrob Agents 27: 553–556.

Dasta JF and Armstrong DK (1988) Variability in aminoglycoside pharmacokinetics in critically ill surgical patients. Crit Care Med 16: 327–330.

Day IP, Goudie J, Nishiki K, et al. (1995) Correlation between in vitro and in vivo models of proconvulsive activity with the carbapenem antibiotics, biapenem, imipenem/cilastatin and meropenem. Toxicol Lett 76: 239–243.

De Gaudio AR and Di Filippo A (2003) What is the role of streptogramins in intensive care? J Chemother 15 Suppl 3: 17–21.

DeHaan RM, Metzler CM, Schellenberg D, et al. (1973) Pharmacokinetic studies of clindamycin phosphate. J Clin Pharmacol 13: 190–209.

Dellinger RP, Levy MM, Carlet JM, et al. (2008) Surviving sepsis campaign: international guidelines for management of severe sepsis and septic shock: 2008. Crit Care Med 36: 296–327.

Di Giantomasso D, May CN, and Bellomo R (2002) Norepinephrine and vital organ blood flow. Intensive Care Med 28: 1804–1809,

Di Giantomasso D, May CN, and Bellomo R (2003) Norepinephrine and vital organ blood flow during experimental hyperdynamic sepsis. Intensive Care Med 29: 1774–1781.

Di Giantomasso D, Bellomo R, and May CN (2005) The haemodynamic and metabolic effects of epinephrine in experimental hyperdynamic septic shock. Intensive Care Med 31: 454–462.

Dong Y, Zhao X, Domagala J, et al. (1999) Effect of fluoroquinolone concentration on selection of resistant mutants of Mycobacterium bovis BCG and Staphylococcus aureus. Antimicrob Agents Chemother 43: 1756–1758.

Drusano GL (2003) Prevention of resistance: a goal for dose selection for antimicrobial agents. Clin Infect Dis 36: S42–S50.

Drusano GL (2004) Antimicrobial pharmacodynamics: critical interactions of 'bug and drug'. Nat Rev Microbiol 2: 289–300.

Duffull SB, Begg EJ, Chambers ST, et al. (1994) Efficacies of different vancomycin dosing regimens against Staphylococcus aureus determined with a dynamic in vitro model. Antimicrob Agents Chemother 38: 2480–2482.

Duffull SB, Kirkpatrick CM, and Begg EJ (1997) Comparison of two Bayesian approaches to dose-individualization for once-daily aminoglycoside regimens. Br J Clin Pharmacol 43: 125–135.

Dvorchik B, Sica D, and Gehr T (2002) Pharmacokinetics and safety of single-dose daptomycin in subjects with graded renal insufficiency and end-stage renal disease. Interscience Conference on Antimicrobial Agents and Chemotherapy, San Diego.

Dvorchik BH, Brazier D, DeBruin MF, et al. (2003) Daptomycin pharmacokinetics and safety following administration of escalating doses once daily to healthy subjects. Antimicrob Agents Chemother 47: 1318–1323.

Elting LS, Rubenstein EB, Kurtin D, et al. (1998) Mississippi mud in the 1990s: risks and outcomes of vancomycin-associated toxicity in general oncology practice. Cancer 83: 2597–2607.

Fantin B, Ebert S, Leggett J, et al. (1991) Factors affecting duration of in-vivo postantibiotic effect for aminoglycosides against gram-negative bacilli. J Antimicrob Chemother 27: 829–836.

Fantin B, Farinotti R, Thabaut A, et al. (1994) Conditions for the emergence of resistance to cefpirome and ceftazidime in experimental endocarditis due to Pseudomonas aeruginosa. J Antimicrob Chemother 33: 563–569.

Fass RJ and Saslaw S (1972) Clindamycin: clinical and laboratory evaluation of parenteral therapy. Am J Med Sci 263: 368–382.

Fink MP, Snydman DR, Niederman MS, et al. (1994) Treatment of severe pneumonia in hospitalized patients: results of a multicenter, randomized, double-blind trial comparing intravenous ciprofloxacin with imipenem-cilastatin. The Severe Pneumonia Study Group. Antimicrob Agents Chemother 38: 547–557.

Firsov AA, Zinner SH, Vostrov SN, et al. (2002) Comparative pharmacodynamics of azithromycin and roxithromycin with S. pyogenes and S. pneumoniae in a model that simulates in vitro pharmacokinetics in human tonsils. J Antimicrob Chemother 49: 113–119.

Firsov AA, Vostrov SN, Lubenko IY, et al. (2003) In vitro pharmacodynamic evaluation of the mutant selection window hypothesis using four fluoroquinolones against Staphylococcus aureus. Antimicrob Agents Chemother 47: 1604–1613.

Firsov AA, Smirnova MV, Lubenko IY, et al. (2006) Testing the mutant selection window hypothesis with Staphylococcus aureus exposed to daptomycin and vancomycin in an in vitro dynamic model. J Antimicrob Chemother 58: 1185–1192.

Fisman DN and Kaye KM (2000) Once daily dosing of aminoglycoside antibiotics. Infect Dis Clin North Am 14: 475–487.

Forrest A, Nix DE, Ballow CH, et al. (1993) Pharmacodynamics of intravenous ciprofloxacin in seriously ill patients. Antimicrob Agents Chemother 37: 1073–1081.

Foulds G, Shepard RM, and Johnson RB (1990) The pharmacokinetics of azithromycin in human serum and tissues. J Antimicrob Chemother 25 Suppl A: 73–82.

Freebairn RC and Lipman J (1993a) Renal replacement therapy for the critically ill – precarious progress. Part II. Technical aspects and clinical application. S Afr J Surg 31: 147–151.

Freebairn RC and Lipman J (1993b) Renal replacement therapy for the critically ill – precarious progress. Part I. Definitions and physiological aspects. S Afr J Surg 31: 114–120.

French G (2003) Safety and tolerability of linezolid. J Antimicrob Chemother 51 Suppl 2: ii45–ii53.

Fry DE (1996) The importance of antibiotic pharmacokinetics in critical illness. Am J Surg 172: 20S–25S.

Fuhs DW, Mann HJ, Kubajak CA, et al. (1988) Intrapatient variation of aminoglycoside pharmacokinetics in critically ill surgery patients. Clin Pharm 7: 207–213.

Garnacho-Montero J, Garcia-Garmendia JL, Barrero-Almodovar A, et al. (2003) Impact of adequate empirical antibiotic therapy on the outcome of patients admitted to the intensive care unit with sepsis. Crit Care Med 31: 2742–2751.

Gattringer R, Urbauer E, Traunmuller F, et al. (2004) Pharmacokinetics of telithromycin in plasma and soft tissues after single-dose administration to healthy volunteers. Antimicrob Agents Chemother 48: 4650–4653.

Gentry-Nielsen MJ, Olsen KM, and Preheim LC (2002) Pharmacodynamic activity and efficacy of line-zolid in a rat model of pneumococcal pneumonia. Antimicrob Agents Chemother 46: 1345–1351.

Georges B, Archambaud M, Saivin S, et al. (1999) Continuous versus intermittent cefepime infu-sion in critical care. [Preliminary results]. Pathol Biol (Paris) 47: 483–485.

Georges B, Conil JM, Cougot P, et al. (2005) Cefepime in critically ill patients: continuous infu-sion vs. an intermittent dosing regimen. Int J Clin Pharmacol Ther 43: 360–369.

Gerson SL, Kaplan SL, Bruss JB, et al. (2002) Hematologic effects of linezolid: summary of clini-cal experience. Antimicrob Agents Chemother 46: 2723–2726.

Gibson TP, Demetriades JL, and Bland JA (1985) Imipenem/cilastatin: pharmacokinetic profile in renal insufficiency. Am J Med 78: 54–61.

Gomez CM, Cordingly JJ, and Palazzo MG (1999) Altered pharmacokinetics of ceftazidime in critically ill patients. Antimicrob Agents Chemother 43: 1798–1802.

Gordon RC, Regamey C, and Kirby WM (1973) Serum protein binding of erythromycin, linco-mycin, and clindamycin. J Pharm Sci 62: 1074–1077.

Gosling P, Sanghera K, and Dickson G (1994) Generalized vascular permeability and pulmonary function in patients following serious trauma. J Trauma 36: 477–481.

Goss TF, Forrest A, Nix DE, et al. (1994) Mathematical examination of dual individualization principles (II): the rate of bacterial eradication at the same area under the inhibitory curve is more rapid for ciprofloxacin than for cefmenoxime. Ann Pharmacother 28: 863–868.

Gous A, Lipman J, Scribante J, et al. (2005) Fluid shifts have no influence on ciprofloxacin pharmacoki-netics in intensive care patients with intra-abdominal sepsis. Int J Antimicrob Agents 26: 50–55.

Gous AG, Dance MD, Lipman J, et al. (1995) Changes in vancomycin pharmacokinetics in criti-cally ill infants. Anaesth Intensive Care 23: 678–682.

Graninger W and Zeitlinger M (2004) Clinical applications of levofloxacin for severe infections. Chemotherapy 50 Suppl 1: 16–21.

Griswold MW, Lomaestro BM, and Briceland LL (1996) Quinupristin-dalfopristin (RP 59500): an injectable streptogramin combination. Am J Health Syst Pharm 53: 2045–2053.

Grocott-Mason RM and Shah AM (1998) Cardiac dysfunction in sepsis: new theories and clinical implications. Intensive Care Med 24: 286–295.

Gudmundsson S, Vogelman B, and Craig WA (1986) The in-vivo postantibiotic effect of imi-penem and other new antimicrobials. J Antimicrob Chemother 18 Suppl E: 67–73.

Gunderson BW, Ross GH, Ibrahim KH, et al. (2001) What do we really know about antibiotic pharmacodynamics. Pharmacotherapy 21: 302–318.

Gwilt PR and Smith RB (1986) Protein binding and pharmacokinetics of lincomycin following intravenous administration of high doses. J Clin Pharmacol 26: 87–90.

Hanes SD, Wood GC, Herring V, et al. (2000) Intermittent and continuous ceftazidime infusion for critically ill trauma patients. Am J Surg 179: 436–440.

Harbarth S, Garbino J, Pugin J, et al. (2003) Inappropriate initial antimicrobial therapy and its effect on survival in a clinical trial of immunomodulating therapy for severe sepsis. Am J Med 115: 529–535.

Hatala R, Dinh TT, and Cook DJ (1997) Single daily dosing of aminoglycosides in immunocom-promised adults: a systematic review. Clin Infect Dis 24: 810–815.

Henderson-Begg SK, Livermore DM, and Hall LM (2006) Effect of subinhibitory concentrations of antibiotics on mutation frequency in Streptococcus pneumoniae. J Antimicrob Chemother 57: 849–854.

Herrera-Gutierrez ME, Seller-Perez G, Banderas-Bravo E, et al. (2007) Replacement of 24-h cre-atinine clearance by 2-h creatinine clearance in intensive care unit patients: a single-center study. Intensive Care Med 33: 1900–1906.

Hoepelman AI, Kieft H, Aoun M, et al. (1993) International comparative study of cefepime and ceftazidime in the treatment of serious bacterial infections. J Antimicrob Chemother 32 Suppl B: 175–186.

Hoffken G, Lode H, Prinzing C, et al. (1985) Pharmacokinetics of ciprofloxacin after oral and parenteral administration. Antimicrob Agents Chemother 27: 375–379.

Hollingsed TC, Harper DJ, Jennings JP, et al. (1993) Aminoglycoside dosing in burn patients using first-dose pharmacokinetics. J Trauma 35: 394–398.

Hugonnet S, Harbarth S, Ferriere K, et al. (2003) Bacteremic sepsis in intensive care: temporal trends in incidence, organ dysfunction, and prognosis. Crit Care Med 31: 390–394.

Hyatt JM and Schentag JJ (2000) Pharmacodynamic modeling of risk factors for ciprofloxacin resistance in Pseudomonas aeruginosa. Infect Control Hosp Epidemiol 21: S9–S11.

Ibrahim EH, Sherman G, Ward S, et al. (2000) The influence of inadequate antimicrobial treatment of bloodstream infections on patient outcomes in the ICU setting. Chest 118: 146–155.

Jacobs MR, Bajaksouzian S, and Appelbaum PC (2003) Telithromycin post-antibiotic and post-antibiotic sub-MIC effects for 10 gram-positive cocci. J Antimicrob Chemother 52: 809–812.

James JK, Palmer SM, Levine DP, et al. (1996) Comparison of conventional dosing versus continuous-infusion vancomycin therapy for patients with suspected or documented gram-positive infections. Antimicrob Agents Chemother 40: 696–700.

Jaruratanasirikul S, Sriwiriyajan S, and Ingviya N (2002) Continuous infusion versus intermittent administration of cefepime in patients with gram-negative bacilli bacteraemia. J Pharm Pharmacol 54: 1693–1696.

Jauregui L, Matzke D, Scott M, et al. (1993) Cefepime as treatment for osteomyelitis and other severe bacterial infections. J Antimicrob Chemother 32 Suppl B: 141–149.

Jones EM (1997) The pharmacokinetics of intravenous ciprofloxacin 400 mg 12 hourly in patients with severe sepsis: the effect of renal function and intra-abdominal disease. J Antimicrob Chemother 40: 121–124.

Joukhadar C, Frossard M, Mayer BX, et al. (2001) Impaired target site penetration of beta-lactams may account for therapeutic failure in patients with septic shock. Crit Care Med 29: 385–391.

Joy MS, Matzke GR, Armstrong DK, et al. (1998a) A primer on continuous renal replacement therapy for critically ill patients. Ann Pharmacother 32: 362–375.

Joy MS, Matzke GR, Frye RF, et al. (1998b) Determinants of vancomycin clearance by continuous venovenous hemofiltration and continuous venovenous hemodialysis. Am J Kidney Dis 31: 1019–1027.

Joynt GM, Lipman J, Gomersall CD, et al. (2001) The pharmacokinetics of once-daily dosing of ceftriaxone in critically ill patients. J Antimicrob Chemother 47: 421–429.

Kapusnik JE, Hackbarth CJ, Chambers HF, et al. (1988) Single, large, daily dosing versus intermittent dosing of tobramycin for treating experimental pseudomonas pneumonia. J Infect Dis 158: 7–12.

Kasbekar N and Acharya PS (2005) Telithromycin: the first ketolide for the treatment of respiratory infections. Am J Health Syst Pharm 62: 905–916.

Kashuba ADM, Nafiziger AN, Drusano GL, et al. (1999) Optimizing aminoglycoside therapy for nosocomial pneumonia caused by gram-negative bacteria. Antimicrob Agents Chemother 43: 623–629.

Kieft H, Hoepelman AI, Knupp CA, et al. (1993) Pharmacokinetics of cefepime in patients with the sepsis syndrome. J Antimicrob Chemother 32 Suppl B: 117–122.

Kim KS (1985) Efficacy of cefmenoxime in experimental Escherichia coli bacteremia and meningitis. Antimicrob Agents Chemother 28: 389–392.

Kirkpatrick CM, Duffull SB, Begg EJ, et al. (2003) The use of a change in gentamicin clearance as an early predictor of gentamicin-induced nephrotoxicity. Ther Drug Monit 25: 623–630.

Kitzes-Cohen R, Farin D, Piva G, et al. (2002) Pharmacokinetics and pharmacodynamics of meropenem in critically ill patients. Int J Antimicrob Agents 19: 105–110.

Klatersky J (1986) Concept of empiric therapy with antibiotic combinations: indications and limits. Am J Med 80: 2–12.

Klepser ME, Patel KB, Nicolau DP, et al. (1998) Comparison of bactericidal activities of intermittent and continuous infusion dosing of vancomycin against methicillin-resistant Staphylococcus aureus and Enterococcus faecalis. Pharmacotherapy 18: 1069–1074.

Knudsen JD, Fuursted K, Raber S, et al. (2000) Pharmacodynamics of glycopeptides in the mouse peritonitis model of Steptococcus pneumoniae or Staphylococcus aureus infection. Antimicrob Agents Chemother 44: 1247–1254.

Knudsen JD, Odenholt I, Erlendsdottir H, et al. (2003) Selection of resistant Streptococcus pneumoniae during penicillin treatment in vitro and in three animal models. Antimicrob Agents Chemother 47: 2499–2506.

Kollef MH, Sherman G, Ward S, et al. (1999) Inadequate antimicrobial treatment of infections: a risk factor for hospital mortality among critically ill patients. Chest 115: 462–474.

Konishi K, Suzuki H, Saruta T, et al. (1991) Removal of imipenem and cilastatin by hemodialysis in patients with end-stage renal failure. Antimicrob Agents Chemother 35: 1616–1620.

Kotapati S, Nicolau DP, Nightingale CH, et al. (2004) Clinical and economic benefits of a meropenem dosage strategy based on pharmacodynamic concepts. Am J Health Syst Pharm 61: 1264–1270.

Krueger WA, Lenhart FP, Neeser G, et al. (2002) Influence of combined intravenous and topical antibiotic prophylaxis on the incidence of infections, organ dysfunctions, and mortality in critically ill surgical patients: a prospective, stratified, randomized, double-blind, placebo-controlled clinical trial. Am J Respir Crit Care Med 166: 1029–1037.

Krueger WA, Bulitta J, Kinzig-Schippers M, et al. (2005) Evaluation by Monte Carlo simulation of the pharmacokinetics of two doses of meropenem administered intermittently or as a continuous infusion in healthy volunteers. Antimicrob Agents Chemother 49: 1881–1889.

Kumar A, Roberts D, Wood KE, et al. (2006) Duration of hypotension before initiation of effective antimicrobial therapy is the critical determinant of survival in human septic shock. Crit Care Med 34: 1589–1596.

Laethem T, De Lepeleire I, McCrea J, et al. (2003) Tissue penetration by ertapenem, a parenteral carbapenem administered once daily, in suction-induced skin blister fluid in healthy young volunteers. Antimicrob Agents Chemother 47: 1439–1442.

LaPlante KL, Rybak MJ, Tsuji B, et al. (2007) Fluoroquinolone resistance in Streptococcus pneumoniae: area under the concentration–time curve/MIC ratio and resistance development with gatifloxacin, gemifloxacin, levofloxacin, and moxifloxacin. Antimicrob Agents Chemother 51: 1315–1320.

Larsson AJ, Walker KJ, Raddatz JK, et al. (1996) The concentration-independent effect of monoexponential and biexponential decay in vancomycin concentrations on the killing of Staphylococcus aureus under aerobic and anaerobic conditions. J Antimicrob Chemother 38: 589–597.

Lavigne JP, Bonnet R, Michaux-Charachon S, et al. (2004) Post-antibiotic and post-beta-lactamase inhibitor effects of ceftazidime plus sulbactam on extended-spectrum beta-lactamase-producing gram-negative bacteria. J Antimicrob Chemother 53: 616–619.

Leggett JE, Fantin B, and Ebert S (1989) Comparative antibiotic dose-effect relations at several dosing intervals in murine pneumonitis and thigh-infection models. J Infect Dis 159: 281–292.

Leroy A, Fillastre JP, Etienne I, et al. (1992) Pharmacokinetics of meropenem in subjects with renal insufficiency. Eur J Clin Pharmacol 42: 535–538.

Lesne-Hulin A, Bourget P, Le Bever H, et al. (1997) Therapeutic monitoring of teicoplanin in a severely burned patient. Ann Fr Anesth Reanim 16: 374–377.

Levey AS, Bosch JP, Lewis JB, et al. (1999) A more accurate method to estimate glomerular filtration rate from serum creatinine: a new prediction equation. Modification of Diet in Renal Disease Study Group. Ann Intern Med 130: 461–470.

Levison ME (1995) Pharmacodynamics of antimicrobial agents. Bactericidal and postantibiotic effects. Infect Dis Clin North Am 9: 483–495.

Levitt DG (2003) The pharmacokinetics of the interstitial space in humans. BMC Clin Pharmacol 3: 3–32.

Lipman J (2005) Is the end-game penetration (of the airway)? Crit Care Med 33: 1654–1655.

Lipman J, Crewe-Brown HH, Saunders GL, et al. (1996) Subtleties of antibiotic dosages – do doses and intervals make a difference in the critically ill? S Afr J Surg 34: 160–162.

Lipman J, Scribante J, Gous AG, et al. (1998) Pharmacokinetic profiles of high-dose intravenous ciprofloxacin in severe sepsis. The Baragwanath Ciprofloxacin Study Group. Antimicrob Agents Chemother 42: 2235–2239.

Lipman J, Gomersall CD, Gin T, et al. (1999a) Continuous infusion ceftazidime in intensive care: a randomized controlled trial. J Antimicrob Chemother 43: 309–311.

Lipman J, Wallis SC, and Rickard C (1999b) Low plasma cefepime levels in critically ill septic patients: pharmacokinetic modeling indicates improved troughs with revised dosing. Antimicrob Agents Chemother 43: 2559–2561.

Lipman J, Wallis SC, Rickard CM, et al. (2001) Low cefpirome levels during twice daily dosing in critically ill septic patients: pharmacokinetic modelling calls for more frequent dosing. Intensive Care Med 27: 363–370.

Lipman J, Gous AG, Mathivha LR, et al. (2002) Ciprofloxacin pharmacokinetic profiles in paediatric sepsis: how much ciprofloxacin is enough? Intensive Care Med 28: 493–500.

Lipman J, Wallis SC, and Boots RJ (2003) Cefepime versus cefpirome: the importance of creatinine clearance. Anesth Analg 97: 1149–1154, Table of contents.

Lode H, Borner K, and Koeppe P (1998) Pharmacodynamics of fluoroquinolones. Clin Infect Dis 27: 33–39.

Lodise TP, Jr., Lomaestro B, and Drusano GL (2007) Piperacillin-tazobactam for Pseudomonas aeruginosa infection: clinical implications of an extended-infusion dosing strategy. Clin Infect Dis 44: 357–363.

Loirat P, Rohan J, Baillet A, et al. (1978) Increased glomerular filtration rate in patients with major burns and its effect on the pharmacokinetics of tobramycin. N Engl J Med 299: 915–919.

Lorente L, Garcia C, Martin M, et al. (2005a) Continuous infusion versus intermittent infusion of ceftazidime for the treatment of pneumonia caused by Pseudomonas aeruginosa. 25th International Symposium on Intensive Care and Emergency Medicine, Brussels, Belgium, Critical Care.

Lorente L, Huidobro S, Martín M, et al. (2005b) Meropenem administration by intermittent infusion versus continuous infusion for the treatment of nosocomial pneumonia. Crit Care 9: P38.

Lorente L, Lorenzo L, Martin MM, et al. (2006) Meropenem by continuous versus intermittent infusion in ventilator-associated pneumonia due to gram-negative bacilli. Ann Pharmacother 40: 219–223.

Lowdin E, Odenholt I, and Cars O (1998) In vitro studies of pharmacodynamic properties of vancomycin against Staphylococcus aureus and Staphylococcus epidermidis. Antimicrob Agents Chemother 42: 2739–2744.

MacArthur RD, Miller M, Albertson T, et al. (2004) Adequacy of early empiric antibiotic treatment and survival in severe sepsis: experience from the MONARCS trial. Clin Infect Dis 38: 284–288.

MacGowan A, Rogers C, and Bowker K (2000) The use of in vitro pharmacodynamic models of infection to optimize fluoroquinolone dosing regimens. J Antimicrob Chemother 46: 163–170.

MacGowan AP (1998) Pharmacodynamics, pharmacokinetics, and therapeutic drug monitoring of glycopeptides. Ther Drug Monit 20: 473–477.

MacGowan AP (2003) Pharmacokinetic and pharmacodynamic profile of linezolid in healthy volunteers and patients with gram-positive infections. J Antimicrob Chemother 51 Suppl 2: ii17–ii25.

MacGowan AP and Bowker KE (1998) Continuous infusion of beta-lactam antibiotics. Clin Pharmacokinet 35: 391–402.

MacKenzie FM and Gould IM (1993) The post-antibiotic effect. J Antimicrob Chemother 32: 519–537.

Mangione A and Schentag JJ (1980) Therapeutic monitoring of aminoglycoside antibiotics: an approach. Ther Drug Monit 2: 159–167.

Mann HJ, Fuhs DW, Awang R, et al. (1987a) Altered aminoglycoside pharmacokinetics in critically ill patients with sepsis. Clin Pharm 6: 148–153.

Mann HJ, Townsend RJ, Fuhs DW, et al. (1987b) Decreased hepatic clearance of clindamycin in critically ill patients with sepsis. Clin Pharm 6: 154–159.

Marik PE (1993) Aminoglycoside volume of distribution and illness severity in critically ill septic patients. Anaesth Intensive Care 21: 172–173.

Marik PE, Havlik I, Monteagudo FS, et al. (1991a) The pharmacokinetic of amikacin in critically ill adult and paediatric patients: comparison of once- versus twice-daily dosing regimens. J Antimicrob Chemother 27 Suppl C: 81–89.

Marik PE, Lipman J, Kobilski S, et al. (1991b) A prospective randomized study comparing once-versus twice-daily amikacin dosing in critically ill adult and paediatric patients. J Antimicrob Chemother 28: 753–764.

Marshall JC (2001) Inflammation, coagulopathy, and the pathogenesis of multiple organ dysfunction syndrome. Crit Care Med 29: S99–S106.

Matzke GR, McGory RW, Halstenson CE, et al. (1984) Pharmacokinetics of vancomycin in patients with various degrees of renal function. Antimicrob Agents Chemother 25: 433–437.

Mazzei T, Surrenti C, Novelli A, et al. (1993) Pharmacokinetics of azithromycin in patients with impaired hepatic function. J Antimicrob Chemother 31 Suppl E: 57–63.

McDonald P, Wetherall B, and Pruul H (1981) Postantibiotic leukocyte enhancement: increased susceptibility of bacteria pretreated with antibiotics to activity of leukocytes. Rev Infect Dis 3: 38–44.

McKindley DS, Boucher BA, Hess MM, et al. (1996) Pharmacokinetics of aztreonam and imipenem in critically ill patients with pneumonia. Pharmacotherapy 16: 924–931.

McNabb JJ, Nightingale CH, Quintiliani R, et al. (2001) Cost-effectiveness of ceftazidime by continuous infusion versus intermittent infusion for nosocomial pneumonia. Pharmacotherapy 21: 549–555.

Meagher AK, Ambrose PG, Grasela TH, et al. (2005a) The pharmacokinetic and pharmacodynamic profile of tigecycline. Clin Infect Dis 41 Suppl 5: S333–S340.

Meagher AK, Ambrose PG, Grasela TH, et al. (2005b) Pharmacokinetic/pharmacodynamic profile for tigecycline – a new glycylcycline antimicrobial agent. Diagn Microbiol Infect Dis 52: 165–171.

MICROMEDEX T. (1974–2005). Micromedex Healthcare Series. DRUGDEX Evaluations, 2005.

MIMS Australia. (2005a). Synercid IV (R), Product Information. MIMS Online Retrieved 18/12/2005, 2005.

MIMS Australia. (2005b). Ciproxin(R) Product Information. MIMS Online Retrieved 14th September, 2005.

Mohr JF, Wanger A, and Rex JH (2004) Pharmacokinetic/pharmacodynamic modeling can help guide targeted antimicrobial therapy for nosocomial gram-negative infections in critically ill patients. Diagn Microbiol Infect Dis 48: 125–130.

Moore RD, Lietman PS, and Smith CR (1987) Clinical response to aminoglycoside therapy: importance of the ratio of peak concentration to minimal inhibitory concentration. J Infect Dis 155: 93–99.

Mouton JW and den Hollander JG (1994) Killing of Pseudomonas aeruginosa during continuous and intermittent infusion of ceftazidime in an in vitro pharmacokinetic model. Antimicrob Agents Chemother 38: 931–936.

Mouton JW and Vinks AA (2005) Pharmacokinetic/pharmacodynamic modelling of antibacterials in vitro and in vivo using bacterial growth and kill kinetics: the minimum inhibitory concentration versus stationary concentration. Clin Pharmacokinet 44: 201–210.

Mouton JW, Vinks AA, and Punt NC (1997) Pharmacokinetic-pharmacodynamic modeling of activity of ceftazidime during continuous and intermittent infusion. Antimicrob Agents Chemother 41: 733–738.

Mouton JW, Touzw DJ, Horrevorts AM, et al. (2000) Comparative pharmacokinetics of the carbapenems: clinical implications. Clin Pharmacokinet 39: 185–201.

Mueller SC, Henkel KO, Neumann J, et al. (1999) Perioperative antibiotic prophylaxis in maxillofacial surgery: penetration of clindamycin into various tissues. J Craniomaxillofac Surg 27: 172–176.

Muller-Serieys C, Andrews J, Vacheron F, et al. (2004) Tissue kinetics of telithromycin, the first ketolide antibacterial. J Antimicrob Chemother 53: 149–157.

Munckhof WJ, Grayson ML, and Turnidge JD (1996) A meta-analysis of studies on the safety and efficacy of aminoglycosides given either once daily or as divided doses. J Antimicrob Chemother 37: 645–663.

Muralidharan G, Micalizzi M, Speth J, et al. (2005) Pharmacokinetics of tigecycline after single and multiple doses in healthy subjects. Antimicrob Agents Chemother 49: 220–229.

Nagar H, Berger SA, Hammar B, et al. (1989) Penetration of clindamycin and metronidazole into the appendix and peritoneal fluid in children. Eur J Clin Pharmacol 37: 209–210.

Nakashima M, Uematsu T, Kosuge K, et al. (1995) Single- and multiple-dose pharmacokinetics of AM-1155, a new 6-fluoro-8-methoxy quinolone, in humans. Antimicrob Agents Chemother 39: 2635–2640.

Namour F, Sultan E, Pascual MH, et al. (2002) Penetration of telithromycin (HMR 3647), a new ketolide antimicrobial, into inflammatory blister fluid following oral administration. J Antimicrob Chemother 49: 1035–1038.

Nguyen M and Chung EP (2005) Telithromycin: the first ketolide antimicrobial. Clin Ther 27: 1144–1163.

Nicolau DP (1998) Optimizing antimicrobial therapy and emerging pathogens. Am J Manag Care 4: S525–S530.

Nicolau DP (2003) Optimizing outcomes with antimicrobial therapy through pharmacodynamic profiling. J Infect Chemother 9: 292–296.

Nicolau DP, Freeman CD, Belliveau PP, et al. (1995) Experience with a once-daily aminoglycoside program administered to 2,184 adult patients. Antimicrob Agents Chemother 39: 650–655.

Nicolau DP, McNabb J, Lacy MK, et al. (2001) Continuous versus intermittent administration of ceftazidime in intensive care unit patients with nosocomial pneumonia. Int J Antimicrob Agents 17: 497–504.

Nix DE, Spivey JM, Norman A, et al. (1992) Dose-ranging pharmacokinetic study of cipro-floxacin after 200-, 300-, and 400-mg intravenous doses. Ann Pharmacother 26: 8–10.

Norrby SR, Newell PA, Faulkner KL, et al. (1995) Safety profile of meropenem: international clinical experience based on the first 3125 patients treated with meropenem. J Antimicrob Chemother 36 Suppl A: 207–223.

Novelli A, Adembri C, Livi P, et al. (2005) Pharmacokinetic evaluation of meropenem and imi-penem in critically ill patients with sepsis. Clin Pharmacokinet 44: 539–549.

Nuytinck HK, Offermans XJ, Kubat K, et al. (1988) Whole-body inflammation in trauma patients. An autopsy study. Arch Surg 123: 1519–1524.

Odenholt I, Lowdin E, and Cars O (2001) Pharmacodynamics of telithromycin in vitro against respiratory tract pathogens. Antimicrob Agents Chemother 45: 23–29.

Olofsson SK and Cars O (2007) Optimizing drug exposure to minimize selection of antibiotic resistance. Clin Infect Dis 45 Suppl 2: S129–S136.

Olofsson SK, Marcusson LL, Komp Lindgren P, et al. (2006) Selection of ciprofloxacin resistance in Escherichia coli in an in vitro kinetic model: relation between drug exposure and mutant prevention concentration. J Antimicrob Chemother 57: 1116–1121.

Olsen KM, Rudis MI, Rebuck JA, et al. (2004) Effect of once-daily dosing vs. multiple daily dosing of tobramycin on enzyme markers of nephrotoxicity. Crit Care Med 32: 1678–1682.

Pankuch GA, Jacobs MR, and Appelbaum PC (2003) Postantibiotic effects of daptomycin against 14 staphylococcal and pneumococcal clinical isolates. Antimicrob Agents Chemother 47: 3012–3014.

Parrillo JE (1993) Pathogenetic mechanisms of septic shock. N Engl J Med 328: 1471–1477.

Parrillo JE, Parker MM, Natanson C, et al. (1990) Septic shock in humans. Advances in the understanding of pathogenesis, cardiovascular dysfunction, and therapy. Ann Intern Med 113: 227–242.

Pea F and Furlanut M (2001) Pharmacokinetic aspects of treating infections in the intensive care unit: focus on drug interactions. Clin Pharmacokinet 40: 833–868.

Pea F, Porreca L, Baraldo M, et al. (2000) High vancomycin dosage regimens required by intensive care unit patients cotreated with drugs to improve haemodynamics following cardiac surgical procedures. J Antimicrob Chemother 45: 329–335.

Peterson LR (2005) Antimicrobial activity and pharmacokinetics/pharmacodynamics of the novel glycylcycline, tigecycline. Diagn Microbiol Infect Dis 52: 163–164.

Petersen PJ, Jacobus NV, Weiss WJ, et al. (1999) In vitro and in vivo antibacterial activities of a novel glycylcycline, the 9-t-butylglycylamido derivative of minocycline (GAR-936). Antimicrob Agents Chemother 43: 738–744.

Pharmacia Australia (2005). Product Information: Gentamicin Injection BP (R), Gentamicin Sulphate, Rydalmere, NSW.

Phelps DJ, Carlton DD, Farrell CA, et al. (1986) Affinity of cephalosporins for beta-lactamases as a factor in antibacterial efficacy. Antimicrob Agents Chemother 29: 845–848.

Piddock LJ and Dalhoff A (1993) Should quinolones be used in the treatment of bacterial infections in neutropenic patients? J Antimicrob Chemother 32: 771–774.

Pinder M, Bellomo R, and Lipman J (2002) Pharmacological principles of antibiotic prescription in the critically ill. Anaesth Intensive Care 30: 134–144.

Piscitelli SC, Danziger LH, and Rodvold KA (1992) Clarithromycin and azithromycin: new macrolide antibiotics. Clin Pharm 11: 137–152.

Pong S, Seto W, Abdolell M, et al. (2005) 12-hour versus 24-hour creatinine clearance in critically ill pediatric patients. Pediatr Res 58: 83–88.

Postier RG, Green SL, Klein SR, et al. (2004) Results of a multicenter, randomized, open-label efficacy and safety study of two doses of tigecycline for complicated skin and skin-structure infections in hospitalized patients. Clin Ther 26: 704–714.

Power BM, Forbes AM, van Heerden PV, et al. (1998) Pharmacokinetics of drugs used in critically ill adults. Clin Pharmacokinet 34: 25–56.

Preston SL, Drusano GL, and Berman AL (1998) Pharmaco-dynamics of levofloxacin: a new paradigm for early clinical trials. JAMA 279: 125–129.

Prins JM, Buller HR, Kuijper EJ, et al. (1993) Once versus thrice daily gentamicin in patients with serious infections. Lancet 341: 335–339.

Projan SJ (2000) Preclinical pharmacology of GAR-936, a novel glycylcycline antibacterial agent. Pharmacotherapy 20: 219S–223S; discussion 224S–228S.

Reed RL, 2nd, Wu AH, Miller-Crotchett P, et al. (1989) Pharmacokinetic monitoring of nephrotoxic antibiotics in surgical intensive care patients. J Trauma 29: 1462–1468; discussion 1468–1470.

Rello J, Sole-Violan J, Sa-Borges M, et al. (2005) Pneumonia caused by oxacillin-resistant Staphylococcus aureus treated with glycopeptides. Crit Care Med 33: 1983–1987.

Reyes N, Skinner R, Kaniga K, et al. (2005) Efficacy of telavancin (TD-6424), a rapidly bactericidal lipoglycopeptide with multiple mechanisms of action, in a murine model of pneumonia induced by methicillin-resistant Staphylococcus aureus. Antimicrob Agents Chemother 49: 4344–4346.

Rice TL (1992) Simplified dosing and monitoring of vancomycin for the burn care clinician. Burns 18: 355–361.

Rice TW and Bernard GR (2005) Therapeutic intervention and targets for sepsis. Annu Rev Med 56: 225–248.

Riley HD, Jr. (1970) Vancomycin and novobiocin. Med Clin North Am 54: 1277–1289.

Rivers E, Nguyen B, Havstad S, et al. (2001) Early goal-directed therapy in the treatment of severe sepsis and septic shock. N Engl J Med 345: 1368–1377.

Roberts G, Ibsen P, and Teglman C (2005) Renal function in elderly patients grossly overestimated by MDRD approach to renal function estimation. Society of Hospital Pharmacists of Australia, 27th Federal Conference, Brisbane, Australia.

Roberts JA, Boots R, Rickard CM, et al. (2007a) Is continuous infusion ceftriaxone better than once-a-day dosing in intensive care? A randomized controlled pilot study. J Antimicrob Chemother 59: 285–291.

Roberts JA, Paratz J, Paratz E, et al. (2007b) Continuous infusion of beta-lactam antibiotics in severe infections: a review of its role. Int J Antimicrob Agents 30: 11–18.

Rodvold KA (2001) Pharmacodynamics of antiinfective therapy: taking what we know to the patient's bedside. Pharmacotherapy 21: 319–330.

Romano S, Fdez de Gatta MM, Calvo MV, et al. (1999) Population pharmacokinetics of amikacin in patients with haematological malignancies. J Antimicrob Chemother 44: 235–242.

Roos JF, Lipman J, and Kirkpatrick CM (2007) Population pharmacokinetics and pharmacodynamics of cefpirome in critically ill patients against gram-negative bacteria. Intensive Care Med 33: 781–788.

Roosendaal R, Bakker-Woudenberg IA, Van den Berghe JC, et al. (1986) Continuous versus intermittent administration of ceftazidime in experimental Klebsiella pneumoniae pneumonia in normal and leukopenic rats. Antimicrob Agents Chemother 30: 403–408.

Roosendaal R, Bakker-Woudenberg IA, van den Berghe-van Raffe M, et al. (1989) Impact of the dosage schedule on the efficacy of ceftazidime, gentamicin and ciprofloxacin in Klebsiella pneumoniae pneumonia and septicemia in leukopenic rats. Eur J Clin Microbiol Infect Dis 8: 878–887.

Ross GH, Wright DH, Hovde LB, et al. (2001) Fluoroquinolone resistance in anaerobic bacteria following exposure to levofloxacin, trovafloxacin, and sparfloxacin in an in vitro pharmacodynamic model. Antimicrob Agents Chemother 45: 2136–2140.

Rovers JP, Ilersich AL, and Einarson TR (1995) Meta-analysis of parenteral clindamycin dosing regimens. Ann Pharmacother 29: 852–858.

Rowland M (1990) Clinical pharmacokinetics of teicoplanin. Clin Pharmacokinet 18: 184–209.

Rubinstein E and Vaughan D (2005) Tigecycline: a novel glycylcycline. Drugs 65: 1317–1336.

Rybak MJ (2006) The pharmacokinetic and pharmacodynamic properties of vancomycin. Clin Infect Dis 42 Suppl 1: S35–S39.

Safdar N, Andes D, and Craig WA (2004) In vivo pharmacodynamic activity of daptomycin. Antimicrob Agents Chemother 48: 63–68.

Sanchez A, Lopez-Herce J, Cueto E, et al. (1999) Teicoplanin pharmacokinetics in critically ill paediatric patients. J Antimicrob Chemother 44: 407–409.

Saunders NJ (1994) Why monitor peak vancomycin concentrations? Lancet 344: 1748–1750.

Schentag JJ (1999) Antimicrobial action and pharmaco-kinetics/pharmacodynamics: the use of AUIC to improve efficacy and avoid resistance. J Chemother 11: 426–439.

Schentag JJ, Smith IL, Swanson DJ, et al. (1984) Role for dual individualization with cefmenoxime. Am J Med 77 Suppl 6A: 43–50.

Schetz M, Ferdinande P, Van den Berghe G, et al. (1995) Pharmacokinetics of continuous renal replacement therapy. Intensive Care Med 21: 612–620.

Schriever CA, Fernandez C, Rodvold KA, et al. (2005) Daptomycin: a novel cyclic lipopeptide antimicrobial. Am J Health Syst Pharm 62: 1145–1158.

Sevillano D, Alou L, Aguilar L, et al. (2006) Azithromycin IV pharmacodynamic parameters predicting Streptococcus pneumoniae killing in epithelial lining fluid versus serum: an in vitro pharmacodynamic simulation. J Antimicrob Chemother 57: 1128–1133.

Shi J, Montay G, Chapel S, et al. (2004) Pharmacokinetics and safety of the ketolide telithromycin in patients with renal impairment. J Clin Pharmacol 44: 234–244.

Smith RP, Baltch AL, Franke MA, et al. (2000) Levofloxacin penetrates human monocytes and enhances intracellular killing of Staphylococcus aureus and Pseudomonas aeruginosa. J Antimicrob Chemother 45: 483–488.

Stalker DJ, Jungbluth GL, Hopkins NK, et al. (2003) Pharmacokinetics and tolerance of single- and multiple-dose oral or intravenous linezolid, an oxazolidinone antibiotic, in healthy volunteers. J Antimicrob Chemother 51: 1239–1246.

Stass H (1999) Distribution and tissue penetration of moxifloxacin. Drugs 58: 229–230.

Stass H, Dalhoff A, Kubitza D, et al. (1998) Pharmacokinetics, safety, and tolerability of ascending single doses of moxifloxacin, a new 8-methoxy quinolone, administered to healthy subjects. Antimicrob Agents Chemother 42: 2060–2065.

Stoeckel K (1981) Pharmacokinetics of Rocephin, a highly active new cephalosporin with an exceptionally long biological half-life. Chemotherapy 27 Suppl 1: 42–46.

Sun HK, Kuti JL, and Nicolau DP (2005) Pharmacodynamics of antimicrobials for the empirical treatment of nosocomial pneumonia: a report from the OPTAMA program. Crit Care Med 33: 2222–2227.

Swabb EA, Singhvi SM, Leitz MA, et al. (1983) Metabolism and pharmacokinetics of aztreonam in healthy subjects. Antimicrob Agents Chemother 24: 394–400.

Tally FP, Zeckel M, Wasilewski MM, et al. (1999) Daptomycin: a novel agent for gram-positive infections. Expert Opin Investig Drugs 8: 1223–1238.

Tam VH, Louie A, Lomaestro BM, et al. (2003) Integration of population pharmacokinetics, a pharmacodynamic target, and microbiologic surveillance data to generate a rational empiric dosing strategy for cefepime against Pseudomonas aeruginosa. Pharmacotherapy 23: 291–295.

Tam VH, Louie A, Deziel MR, et al. (2005) Bacterial-population responses to drug-selective pressure: examination of garenoxacin's effect on Pseudomonas aeruginosa. J Infect Dis 192: 420–428.

Tauber MG, Zak O, Scheld WM, et al. (1984) The postantibiotic effect in the treatment of experimental meningitis caused by Streptococcus pneumoniae in rabbits. J Infect Dis 149: 575–583.

Tessier PR, Nicolau DP, Onyeji CO, et al. (1999) Pharmacodynamics of intermittent- and continuous-infusion cefepime alone and in combination with once-daily tobramycin against Pseudomonas aeruginosa in an in vitro infection model. Chemotherapy 45: 284–295.

Thalhammer F, Traunmuller F, El Menyawi I, et al. (1999) Continuous infusion versus intermittent administration of meropenem in critically ill patients. J Antimicrob Chemother 43: 523–527.

Therapeutic Guidelines Antibiotic. (2006). Therapeutic Guidelines Limited, Melbourne.

Thomas JK, Forrest A, Bhavani SM, et al. (1998) Pharmaco-dynamic evaluation of factors associated with the development of bacterial resistance in acutely ill patients during therapy. Antimicrob Agents Chemother 42: 521–527.

Thorburn CE, Molesworth SJ, Sutherland R, et al. (1996) Postantibiotic and post-beta-lactamase inhibitor effects of amoxicillin plus clavulanate. Antimicrob Agents Chemother 40: 2796–2801.

Townsend PL, Fink MP, Stein KL, et al. (1989) Aminoglycoside pharmacokinetics: dosage requirements and nephrotoxicity in trauma patients. Crit Care Med 17: 154–157.

Triginer C, Izquierdo I, Fernandez R, et al. (1990) Gentamicin volume of distribution in critically ill septic patients. Intensive Care Med 16: 303–306.

Trotman RL, Williamson JC, Shoemaker DM, et al. (2005) Antibiotic dosing in critically ill adult patients receiving continuous renal replacement therapy. Clin Infect Dis 41: 1159–1166.

Turnidge J (1998a) Pharmcokinetics and pharmacodynamics of fluoroquinolones. Drugs 58: 29–36.

Turnidge JD (1998b) The pharmacodynamics of beta-lactams. Clin Infect Dis 27: 10–22.

Turnidge J (1999) Fusidic acid pharmacology, pharmacokinetics and pharmacodynamics. Int J Antimicrob Agents 12 Suppl 2: S23–S34.

Valles J, Rello J, Ochagavia A, et al. (2003) Community-acquired bloodstream infection in critically ill adult patients: impact of shock and inappropriate antibiotic therapy on survival. Chest 123: 1615–1624.

Van der Auwera P, Meunier F, Ibrahim S, et al. (1991) Pharmacodynamic parameters and toxicity of netilmicin (6 milligrams/kilogram/day) given once daily or in three divided doses to cancer patients with urinary tract infection. Antimicrob Agents Chemother 35: 640–647.

van der Poll T (2001) Immunotherapy of sepsis. Lancet Infect Dis 1: 165–174.

Viale P and Pea F (2003) What is the role of fluoroquinolones in intensive care? J Chemother 15 Suppl 3: 5–10.

Vogelman BS and Craig WA (1985) Postantibiotic effects. J Antimicrob Chemother 15 Suppl A: 37–46.

Vogelman B and Craig WA (1986) Kinetics of antimicrobial activity. J Pediatr 108: 835–840.

Vogelman B, Gudmundsson S, Leggett J, et al. (1988) Correlation of antimicrobial pharmacokinetic parameters with therapeutic efficacy in an animal model. J Infect Dis 158: 831–847.

Walstad RA, Aanderud L, and Thurmann-Nielsen E (1988) Pharmacokinetics and tissue concentrations of ceftazidime in burn patients. Eur J Clin Pharmacol 35: 543–549.

Weinbren MJ (1999) Pharmacokinetics of antibiotics in burn patients. J Antimicrob Chemother 44: 319–327.

Wells M and Lipman J (1997a) Measurements of glomerular filtration in the intensive care unit are only a rough guide to renal function. S Afr J Surg 35: 20–23.

Wells M and Lipman J (1997b) Pitfalls in the prediction of renal function in the intensive care unit. A review. S Afr J Surg 35: 16–19.

Wilson AP (2000) Clinical pharmacokinetics of teicoplanin. Clin Pharmacokinet 39: 167–183.

Wise R, Gee T, Andrews JM, et al. (2002) Pharmacokinetics and inflammatory fluid penetration of intravenous daptomycin in volunteers. Antimicrob Agents Chemother 46: 31–33.

Woodworth JR, Nyhart EH, Jr., Brier GL, et al. (1992) Single-dose pharmacokinetics and antibacterial activity of daptomycin, a new lipopeptide antibiotic, in healthy volunteers. Antimicrob Agents Chemother 36: 318–325.

Wysocki M, Delatour F, Faurisson F, et al. (2001) Continuous versus intermittent infusion of vancomycin in severe Staphylococcal infections: prospective multicenter randomized study.
Antimicrob Agents Chemother 45: 2460–2467.

Xiong YQ, Caillon J, Kergueris MF, et al. (1997) Adaptive resistance of Pseudomonas aeruginosa
induced by aminoglycosides and killing kinetics in a rabbit endocarditis model. Antimicrob
Agents Chemother 41: 823–826.

Yoshida T, Homma K, Azami K, et al. (1993) Pharmacokinetics of meropenem in experimentally
burned rats. J Dermatol 20: 208–213.

Young RJ, Lipman J, Gin T, et al. (1997) Intermittent bolus dosing of ceftazidime in critically ill
patients. J Antimicrob Chemother 40: 269–273.

Zaske DE, Sawchuk RJ, Gerding DN, et al. (1976) Increased dosage requirements of gentamicin
in burn patients. J Trauma 16: 824–828.

Zaske DE, Cipolle RJ, and Strate RJ (1980) Gentamicin dosage requirements: wide interpatient
variations in 242 surgery patients with normal renal function. Surgery 87: 164–169.

Zhanel GG and Ariano RE (1992) Once daily aminoglycoside dosing: maintained efficacy with
reduced nephrotoxicity? Ren Fail 14: 1–9.

Zhao X and Drlica K (2001) Restricting the selection of antibiotic-resistant mutants: a general
strategy derived from fluoroquinolone studies. Clin Infect Dis 33 Suppl 3: S147–S156.

Zhou J, Dong Y, Zhao X, et al. (2000) Selection of antibiotic-resistant bacterial mutants: allelic
diversity among fluoroquinolone-resistant mutations. J Infect Dis 182: 517–525.

Zinner SH, Lubenko IY, Gilbert D, et al. (2003) Emergence of resistant Streptococcus pneumoniae
in an in vitro dynamic model that simulates moxifloxacin concentrations inside and outside the
mutant selection window: related changes in susceptibility, resistance frequency and bacterial
killing. J Antimicrob Chemother 52: 616–622.

Zuckerman JM (2004) Macrolides and ketolides: azithromycin, clarithromycin, telithromycin.
Infect Dis Clin North Am 18: 621–649.

Index